Percutaneous Vertebroplasty

Springer
New York
Berlin
Heidelberg
Barcelona
Hong Kong
London
Milan
Paris
Singapore
Tokyo

John M. Mathis, MD, MSc
Department of Radiology, Lewis-Gale Medical Center, Salem,
Virginia, USA

Hervé Deramond, MD
Service de Radiologie A, Centre Hospitalier Universitaire d'Amiens,
Amiens, France

Stephen M. Belkoff, PhD
Departments of Orthopaedic Surgery and Mechanical Engineering,
The Johns Hopkins University, Baltimore, Maryland, USA

Editors

Percutaneous Vertebroplasty

With 162 Illustrations

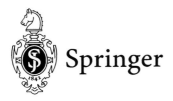 Springer

John M. Mathis, MD, MSc
Department of Radiology
Lewis-Gale Medical Center
Salem, VA 24153, USA
jmathis@rev.net

Hervé Deramond, MD
Service de Radiologie A
Centre Hospitalier
  Universitaire d'Amiens
80054 Amiens, France
deramond.herve@chu-amiens.fr

Stephen M. Belkoff, PhD
Departments of Orthopaedic
  Surgery and Mechanical
  Engineering
The Johns Hopkins University
Baltimore, MD 21224, USA
sbelkoff@jhmi.edu

Library of Congress Cataloging-in-Publication Data
Percutaneous vertebroplasty / editors, John M. Mathis, Hervé Deramond, Stephen M. Belkoff.
    p. ; cm.
  Includes bibliographical references and index.
  ISBN 0-387-95306-X (h/c : alk. paper)
  1. Spine—Surgery. 2. Spine—Fractures. 3. Bone cements. 4. Fracture fixation. I. Mathis, John M.
II. Deramond, Hervé. III. Belkoff, Stephen M.
    [DNLM: 1. Spinal Fractures—surgery. 2. Bone Cements—therapeutic use.
3. Fracture Fixation, Internal—methods. WE 725 P429 2002]
  RD768.P45 2002
  617.5'6059—dc21   2001049252

Printed on acid-free paper.

Production coordinated by Chernow Editorial Services, Inc., and managed by Lesley Poliner; manufacturing su-
pervised by Jeffrey Taub.
Typeset by Matrix Publishing Services, Inc., York, PA.
Printed and bound by Maple-Vail Book Manufacturing Group, York, PA.
Printed in the United States of America.

9 8 7 6 5 4 3 2 1

ISBN 0-387-95306-X   SPIN 10839710

Springer-Verlag   New York Berlin Heidelberg
A member of BertelsmannSpringer Science+Business Media GmbH

Preface

The pain associated with compression fractures of vertebra in the spine has been a relentless problem for patients, their families, and the physicians who treat them. This problem affects a huge population of patients worldwide and, until the conceptualization and introduction of percutaneous vertebroplasty, produced long-term pain and disability. Available therapies were limited to bed rest, analgesics, and external bracing. These were generally slow to relieve the pain. The protracted pain resulted in restricted activities of daily living and often began a progressive spiral of declining independence and loss of self-esteem.

We have been fortunate to be associated with percutaneous vertebroplasty since its beginning in each of our separate geographic areas and professional circles. The observed efficacy of the procedure, along with its low complication rates, has driven us to research the scientific effects of percutaneous bone augmentation, as well as the materials and their shortcomings. In addition, our faith in this procedure has led us to teach our physician colleagues the technical aspects of percutaneous vertebroplasty in courses in Europe and the United States. This process has helped move percutaneous vertebroplasty from an experimental procedure to its present position as a developing standard of care for the treatment of pain resulting from spinal compression fractures.

This book is an extension of our efforts to pass along information that we have accumulated during our educational and scientific journey in the study of percutaneous vertebroplasty.

Our work represents the first written compilation of an up-to-date summary of this information. It is presented here in hopes that our students and colleagues will rapidly gain a high level of proficiency in performing percutaneous vertebroplasty and successfully avoid the potential pitfalls and complications along the way.

JOHN M. MATHIS, MD, MSc
HERVÉ DERAMOND, MD
STEPHEN M. BELKOFF, PhD

Contents

Preface v
Contributors ix

Chapter 1   Introduction: History and Early Development . . .   1
             JOHN M. MATHIS, STEPHEN M. BELKOFF,
             AND HERVÉ DERAMOND

Chapter 2   Spine Anatomy   7
             A. ORLANDO ORTIZ AND HERVÉ DERAMOND

Chapter 3   Osteoporosis: Medical and Surgical Options   25
             ABRAHAM M. OBUCHOWSKI, ALEKSANDAR CURCIN,
             AND JOHN P. KOSTUIK

Chapter 4   Patient Evaluation and Selection   41
             M.J.B. STALLMEYER AND GREGG H. ZOARSKI

Chapter 5   Biomechanical Considerations   61
             STEPHEN M. BELKOFF

Chapter 6   Procedural Techniques and Materials:
             Tumors and Osteoporotic Fractures   81
             JOHN M. MATHIS

Chapter 7   Balloon Kyphoplasty   109
             WADE H. WONG, WAYNE J. OLAN,
             AND STEPHEN M. BELKOFF

Chapter 8   Tumors

Part I   Metastatic Tumors 125
HERVÉ DERAMOND, CLAUDE DEPRIESTER,
AND JACQUES CHIRAS

Part II   Multiple Myeloma 134
ANNE COTTEN, NATHALIE BOUTRY,
AND BERNARD CORTET

Part III   Benign Tumors 138
HERVÉ DERAMOND, ANNE COTTEN,
AND CLAUDE DEPRIESTER

Chapter 9   Extreme Vertebroplasty: Techniques for
Treating Difficult Lesions 155
JOHN D. BARR AND JOHN M. MATHIS

Chapter 10   Complications 165
HERVÉ DERAMOND, JACQUES E. DION,
AND JACQUES CHIRAS

Chapter 11   Starting a Clinical Practice 175
WAYNE J. OLAN AND JOHN M. MATHIS

Chapter 12   Future Directions: Challenges and
Research Opportunities 181
JOHN M. MATHIS, STEPHEN M. BELKOFF,
AND HERVÉ DERAMOND

List of Abbreviations 195
Appendix I: Standard for the Performance of
Percutaneous Vertebroplasty 197
Index 213

Contributors

John D. Barr, MD
Interventional Neuroradiology and Neuroangiography, Baptist
Memorial Hospitals, Memphis, TN 38120, USA.
e-mail: neuroraddoc@hotmail.com

Stephen M. Belkoff, PhD
Departments of Orthopaedic Surgery and Mechanical Engineering,
The Johns Hopkins University, Baltimore, MD 21224, USA.
e-mail: sbelkoff@jhmi.edu

Nathalie Boutry, MD
Service de Radiologie Osteo-articulaire, Hôpital Roger Salengro,
Centre Hospitalier Universitaire de Lille, 59000 Lille, France

Jacques Chiras, MD
Departement de Neuroradiologie Charcot, Groupe Hospitalier la
Pitiè Salpétrière, 75651 Paris 13, France.
e-mail: jaques.chiras@psl.ap-hop-paris.fr

Bernard Cortet, MD
Service de Rhumatologie, Hôpital Roger Salengro, Centre
Hospitalier Universitaire de Lille, 59000 Lille, France

Anne Cotten, MD
Service de Radiologie Osteo-articulaire, Hôpital Roger Salengro,
Centre Hospitalier Universitaire de Lille, 59000 Lille, France

Aleksandar Curcin, MD
Orthopaedic Specialty Center, Baltimore, MD 21209, and
Department of Orthopaedic Surgery, University of Maryland,
Baltimore, MD 21201, USA. e-mail: acurcin@mdorthoteam.com

CLAUDE DEPRIESTER, MD
Service de Radiologie A, Centre Hospitalier Universitaire
d'Amiens, 80054 Amiens, France

HERVÉ DERAMOND, MD
Service de Radiologie A, Centre Hospitalier Universitaire
d'Amiens, 80054 Amiens, France.
e-mail: deramond.herve@chu-amiens.fr

JACQUES E. DION, MD, FRCP(C)
Department of Radiology, Emory University Hospital, Atlanta, GA
30322, USA. e-mail: jacques_dion@emoryhealthcare.org

JOHN P. KOSTUIK, MD
Department of Orthopaedic Surgery, The Johns Hopkins
Outpatient Center, Baltimore, MD 21287, USA.
e-mail: hkowalo@jhmi.edu

JOHN M. MATHIS, MD, MSc
Department of Radiology, Lewis-Gale Medical Center, Salem, VA
24153, USA. e-mail: jmathis@rev.net

ABRAHAM M. OBUCHOWSKI, MD
Department of Diagnostic Radiology, University of Maryland
Medical System, Baltimore, MD 21201, USA.
email: aobuchowski@umm.edu

WAYNE J. OLAN, MD
Department of Radiology, Suburban Hospital, Bethesda, MD
20814, and Department of Radiology, The George Washington
University Medical Center, Washington, DC 20037, USA.
e-mail: w.olanmd@suburbanhospital.org

A. ORLANDO ORTIZ, MD, MBA
Department of Radiology, Winthrop-University Hospital, Mineola,
NY 11501, USA. email: oortiz@winthrop.org

M.J.B. STALLMEYER, MD, PhD
Department of Radiology, University of Maryland, Baltimore, MD
21201, USA. e-mail: bstallmeyer@umm.edu

WADE H. WONG, DO
Department of Radiology, University of California San Diego
Medical Center, and Department of Radiology, Thornton Hospital,
La Jolla, CA 92037, USA. e-mail: cott@ucsd.edu

GREGG H. ZOARSKI, MD
Departments of Radiology and Neurosurgery, University of
Maryland, Baltimore, MD 21201, USA. e-mail: gzoarski@umm.edu

1

Introduction: History and Early Development

John M. Mathis, Stephen M. Belkoff, and Hervé Deramond

For several decades, vertebroplasty has been performed as an open procedure to augment the purchase of pedicle screws for spinal instrumentation[1] and to fill voids resulting from tumor resection.[2–5] The procedure introduces bone graft or acrylic cement into vertebral bodies to mechanically augment their structural integrity.[2–4,6–12] In some cases, however, the risk of an open procedure is not indicated. It was one such case that served as the impetus for the development of percutaneous vertebroplasty (PV). Percutaneous vertebroplasty achieves the benefits of vertebroplasty without the morbidity associated with an open procedure. Vertebral augmentation is accomplished by injecting polymethylmethacrylate (PMMA) cement into a vertebral body via a percutaneously placed cannula. The procedure was first performed in 1984 by Galibert and Deramond in the Department of Radiology of the University Hospital of Amiens, France,[13]on a woman, aged 54, who had complained of severe cervical pain for several years. In 1979 plain radiographs of her cervical spine indicated normal findings, but in 1984, when she presented with unbearable pain associated with a severe radiculopathy localized to the C2 nerve root, plain radiographs showed a large vertebral hemangioma (VH) involving the entire C2 vertebra. An axial computed tomography (CT) scan confirmed epidural extension of the disease. A C2 laminectomy was first performed and the epidural component was excised. To obtain structural reinforcement of the C2 vertebral body, it was decided that cement would be injected percutaneously. A 15-gauge needle was inserted into the C2 verte-

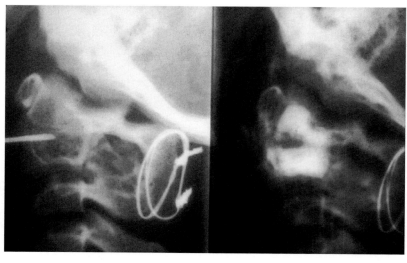

Figure 1-1. The first PV case. (A) Lateral view of C2 with a cannula in place in the VH cavity. (B) Lateral view of C2 after PMMA injection, which resulted in complete pain resolution for this patient.

bral body via an anterolateral approach (Fig. 1-1A). The amount of PMMA injected, calculated on the basis of a transosseous venogram, was 3 mL (Fig. 1-1B). The patient experienced complete pain relief. The results of the procedure were so impressive that the procedure was subsequently used for six other patients. A report describing the outcomes was published in 1987.[13]

The experience gained from those patients, and from some experimental work conducted on fresh cadaveric vertebral bodies, helped establish the main technical points of the procedure.[13–15] These technical points include the use of large-bore (10-gauge) needles in the thoracic and lumbar spine and smaller bore (15-gauge) needles in the cervical spine and the addition of tantalum to the PMMA cement to facilitate fluoroscopic visualization of the distribution of the cement during injection. Early in the clinical experience, a posterolateral approach for the needles was used in the thoracic spine, but, after cement leakage along the track of the needle induced a case of intercostal radiculopathy, a transpedicular needle approach was developed. With the transpedicular approach, the needle passes through the pedicle into the vertebral body, resulting in a lower risk of cement discharging posteriorly along the needle track.

Inspired by the success of the initial PV cases, clinicians from the neuroradiological and neurosurgical teams of the University Hospital in Lyons, France,[16,17] used a slightly modified technique (18-gauge needles) to inject PMMA into the weakened vertebral bodies of seven patients: four with osteoporotic vertebral compression fractures (VCFs), two with VHs, and one with spinal metastasis. The clinicians reported good (one patient) to excellent (six patients) pain relief in these seven initial patients.[16]

In the early 1990s, PV (using Deramond's paradigm) was introduced into clinical practice in the United States via the University of Virginia.[18] Since that time, PV has become a more commonly used method for treating painful vertebral lesions. The European experience has predominantly focused on treating pain related to tumor involvement (both benign and malignant),[13,19–22] whereas the U.S. experience has focused on treating painful osteoporotic VCFs. This continental distinction has become blurred as clinicians on both sides of the Atlantic have responded to changing patient demographics (e.g., increased longevity, increased incidence of osteoporosis, increased numbers of patients surviving cancer—all of whom have higher risks of VCFs).

Severe pain associated with VCF is a very common medical problem; it affects between 700,000 and 1,000,000 patients every year in the United States alone.[23–25] The disease demographics are similar in Europe. Most of these fractures are the result of bone mineral loss due to primary osteoporosis (occurring naturally with age). However, an increasing number of fractures also result from secondary osteoporosis caused by therapeutic drugs such as catabolic steroids, anticonvulsants, cancer chemotherapy, and heparin.[26]

Until the introduction of PV, there were few treatment options other than bed rest and pain management for osteoporotic VCFs. The reportedly immediate and lasting pain relief attained with PV is quickly making the procedure an accepted treatment for osteoporotic VCFs and is challenging the standard medical treatment of bed rest and analgesics. Similarly, because patients with metastatic lesions are surviving longer, there is an increased demand to improve their quality of life and provide mobility during the end stages of their disease. In cases of spinal metastases, PV reportedly relieves pain and structurally augments vertebral bodies compromised by osteolytic lesions, providing some palliation and allowing the patient to continue with weight-bearing activities of daily living.

Thus, it is not surprising that PV has quickly become a popular technique and that the demand for information regarding the procedure is large. Because the procedure is relatively new, the availability of information regarding the procedure has not kept up with the demand. This book functions as a first step in filling that information void by presenting the state of the art of current PV and discussing areas of research that need to be addressed to advance its practice.

References

1. Kostuik JP, Errico TJ, Gleason TF. Techniques of internal fixation for degenerative conditions of the lumbar spine. *Clin Orthop* 1986; 203: 219–231.
2. Cybulski GR. Methods of surgical stabilization for metastatic disease of the spine. *Neurosurgery* 1989; 25(2):240–252.
3. Alleyne CH, Jr, Rodts GE, Jr, Haid RW. Corpectomy and stabilization with methylmethacrylate in patients with metastatic disease of the spine: a technical note. *J Spinal Disord* 1995; 8(6):439–443.
4. Sundaresan N, Galicich JH, Lane JM, et al. Treatment of neoplastic epidural cord compression by vertebral body resection and stabilization. *J Neurosurg* 1985; 63(5):676–684.
5. Scoville WB, Palmer AH, Samra K, et al. The use of acrylic plastic for vertebral replacement or fixation in metastatic disease of the spine. Technical note. *J Neurosurg* 1967; 27(3):274–279.
6. Cortet B, Cotten A, Deprez X, et al. [Value of vertebroplasty combined with surgical decompression in the treatment of aggressive spinal angioma. Apropos of 3 cases.] *Rev Rhum Ed Fr* 1994; 61(1): 16–22.
7. Harrington KD. Anterior decompression and stabilization of the spine as a treatment for vertebral collapse and spinal cord compression from metastatic malignancy. *Clin Orthop* 1988; 233:177–197.
8. Harrington KD, Sim FH, Enis JE, et al. Methylmethacrylate as an adjunct in internal fixation of pathological fractures. Experience with three hundred and seventy-five cases. *J Bone Joint Surg* 1976; 58A(8):1047–1055.
9. Mavian GZ, Okulski CJ. Double fixation of metastatic lesions of the lumbar and cervical vertebral bodies utilizing methylmethacrylate compound: Report of a case and review of a series of cases. *J Am Osteopath Assoc* 1986; 86(3):153–157.
10. O'Donnell RJ, Springfield DS, Motwani HK, et al. Recurrence of giant-cell tumors of the long bones after curettage and packing with cement. *J Bone Joint Surg* 1994; 76A(12):1827–1833.
11. Persson BM, Ekelund L, Lovdahl R, et al. Favourable results of acrylic cementation for giant cell tumors. *Acta Orthop Scand* 1984; 55(2):209–214.
12. Knight G. Paraspinal acrylic inlays in the treatment of cervical and lumbar spondylosis and other conditions. *Lancet* 1959; (ii):147–179.
13. Galibert P, Deramond H, Rosat P, et al. [Preliminary note on the treatment of vertebral angioma by percutaneous acrylic vertebroplasty.] *Neurochirurgie* 1987; 33(2):166–168.
14. Deramond H, Darrason R, Galibert P. [Percutaneous vertebroplasty with acrylic cement in the treatment of aggressive spinal angiomas.] *Rachis* 1989; 1(2):143–153.
15. Darrason R. Place de la vertebroplastie percutanée acrylique dans le traitement des hemangiomes vertebraux agressifs. Doctoral thesis (medicine). Université de Picardie; October 26, 1988.
16. Lapras C, Mottolese C, Deruty R, et al. [Percutaneous injection of methyl-methacrylate in osteoporosis and severe vertebral osteolysis (Galibert's technic).] *Ann Chir* 1989; 43(5):371–376.

17. Bascoulergue Y, Duquesnel J, Leclercq R, et al. Percutaneous injection of methyl methacrylate in the vertebral body for the treatment of various diseases: percutaneous vertebroplasty [abstract]. *Radiology* 1988; 169P:372.

18. Jensen ME, Evans AJ, Mathis JM, et al. Percutaneous polymethyl-methacrylate vertebroplasty in the treatment of osteoporotic vertebral body compression fractures: technical aspects. *Am J Neuroradiol* 1997; 18(10):1897–1904.

19. Cotten A, Dewatre F, Cortet B, et al. Percutaneous vertebroplasty for osteolytic metastases and myeloma: effects of the percentage of lesion filling and the leakage of methyl methacrylate at clinical follow-up. *Radiology* 1996; 200(2):525–530.

20. Kaemmerlen P, Thiesse P, Jonas P, et al. Percutaneous injection of orthopedic cement in metastatic vertebral lesions [letter]. *N Engl J Med* 1989; 321(2):121.

21. Kaemmerlen P, Thiesse P, Bouvard H, et al. [Percutaneous vertebroplasty in the treatment of metastases. Technic and results.] *J Radiol* 1989; 70(10):557–562.

22. Weill A, Chiras J, Simon JM, et al. Spinal metastases: indications for and results of percutaneous injection of acrylic surgical cement. *Radiology* 1996; 199(1):241–247.

23. Melton LJ, III. Epidemiology of spinal osteoporosis. *Spine* 1997; 22(24 suppl):2S–11S.

24. Melton LJ, Kan SH, Wahner HW, et al. Lifetime fracture risk: an approach to hip fracture risk assessment based on bone mineral density and age. *J Clin Epidemiol* 1988; 41(10):985–994.

25. Kanis JA, Johnell O. The burden of osteoporosis. *J Endocrinol Invest* 1999; 22(8):583–588.

26. Miller KK, Klibanski A. Clinical review 106: amenorrheic bone loss. *J Clin Endocrinol Metab* 1999; 84(6):1775–1783.

2

Spine Anatomy

A. Orlando Ortiz and Hervé Deramond

The approach to spinal surgery, as for percutaneous vertebro-plasty (PV), is often defined in terms of the trajectories determined by various spinal and paraspinal anatomical structures such as the spinal canal, paravertebral soft tissues, and osseous anatomy. There are two basic approaches to each of the three spinal areas: lumbar spine, transpedicular and posterolateral approaches; thoracic spine, transpedicular and parapedicular approaches; and cervical spine, anterolateral and (rarely) transoral approaches. This chapter addresses the anatomic landmarks pertinent to those approaches.

Osseous Anatomy

Lumbar Vertebrae

There are five lumbar vertebrae, and their pedicles are larger than those of the thoracic and cervical vertebrae. For this reason, the transpedicular approach (Fig. 2-1) is the most often used for PV in the lumbar region. L1 and L2 are taller dorsally; L4 and L5 are taller ventrally. L3 varies in height with respect to its ventral and dorsal aspects.[1,2] These variations define the lordosis commonly found in the lumbar area. The lumbar spinal canal has a relatively triangular shape, and the neural foramina are directed transversally. The pedicle angles of attachment to the vertebral body (as measured in the ventral-to-dorsal, i.e., anteroposterior [AP], plane) from L5 to L1 vary widely. The largest angle appears in L5, rapidly diminishing to L1 (Fig. 2-2). The pedicles of the lumbar spine are usually well seen as oval structures on an AP

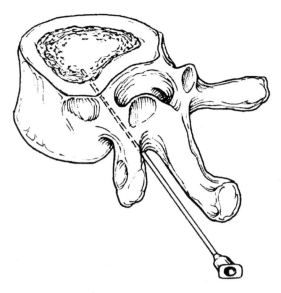

Figure 2-1. Oblique view of the transpedicular approach.

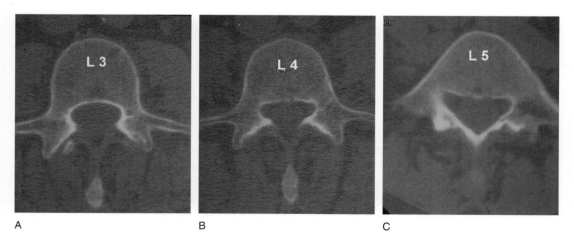

A   B   C

Figure 2-2. The angle of the pedicles increases from L1 to L5, as shown by axial CT scans of the L3 (A), L4 (B), and L5 (C) levels.

fluoroscopic view. The pedicle length creates an oval tunnel of bone that connects the posterior neural arch with the vertebral body.

Thoracic Vertebrae

Thoracic vertebral bodies increase in size from superior to caudal locations. They are slightly taller dorsally than ventrally. In addition to possessing articular facets, these vertebrae have costal facets, which articulate with the ribs. The medial rib end articulates with the vertebra above and the one below via demifacets. These articulations are at the anterolateral aspects of the pedicles. The rib also articulates with the lateral aspect of the transverse process. The close relation between the rib and the transverse process creates the parapedicular route as an alternative for needle placement (Fig. 2-3).[3]

The thoracic pedicles are oriented completely in the ventral-to-dorsal (AP) plane with respect to the vertebral body. The pedicles are smaller than those in the lumbar spine, decreasing in size from T12 through T4.

Cervical Vertebrae

A typical cervical vertebra (C3-C6) consists of a small but broad vertebral body. The pedicle's short height and small AP diameter present a poor target for vertebral access compared to the pedicles of the lumbar and thoracic region.

Size and Orientation of Pedicles

The size and orientation of pedicles are important factors to consider, not only for the performance of transpedicular PV, but also for the design and modification of PV devices. The occurrence of potential complications involving the pedicle, such as pedicle fracture, can be decreased with an appropriate preprocedure evaluation and understanding of pedicle anatomy. Variations in pedicle diameter and the presence of occasional pedicle abnormalities may present a risk to needle placement (e.g., pedicular thinning is an anatomic variant that can occur in the thoracic or lumbar spine). Correct PV needle placement requires the use of a correct entry point on the posterior vertebral cortex.

The vertebral pedicle is a complex three-dimensional cylindroid structure that consists of a thin shell of compact bone, which surrounds a much larger center that is filled with cancellous bone.[4] The superior pedicular cortex has approximately the same thickness as the inferior cortex, except in the midthoracic spine where the superior cortex is thicker.[4] The medial cortex of the pedicle is two to three times thicker than the lateral cortex

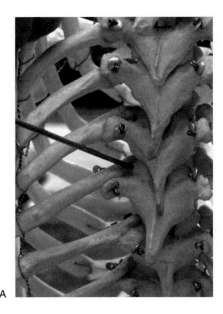

A

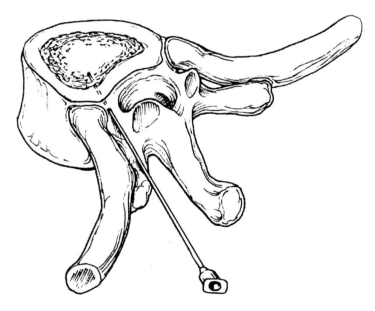

B

Figure 2-3. Parapedicular approach: (A) model of the spine showing needle placement in the thoracic spine and (B) line drawing showing oblique view.

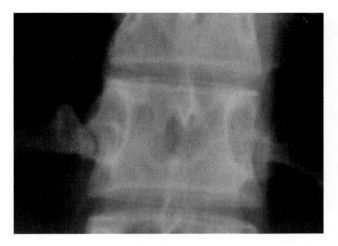

Figure 2-4. Close-up view of frontal projection of thoracic spine shows the relatively thicker medial cortex of the pedicle.

(Fig. 2-4).[4] More than two thirds of fixation-screw-related fractures involve the lateral pedicle wall.[5]

Important factors that should be considered when evaluating a given pedicle are the pedicle size (width, height, and length) and the pedicle angle relative to the vertebral body. Pedicle size is measured at the narrowest point of the pedicle isthmus. The radiographic image of the oval pedicle corresponds to the narrow waist of the pedicle.[6] The pedicle length is measured from the pediculolaminar junction to the posterior vertebral body. The pedicle orientation is described in two planes; the transverse angle is formed between an oblique line drawn through the center of the pedicle axis and a line drawn parallel to the midline at the spinous process, and the sagittal angle is formed between a line drawn through the pedicle axis and either the superior or inferior border of the vertebral body or a line drawn parallel to the vertebral body equator. The pedicle size tends to increase from T4 to L5 (Fig. 2-5).[5]

The large, but short lumbar pedicles arise from the upper lateral portion of the vertebral body. The upper two vertebrae (L1 and L2) are transitional to the thoracic region, and each pedicle is approximately 15 mm high and 8 mm wide.[7] The lower two vertebrae (L4 and L5) are transitional toward the sacrum, and the pedicle of L5 is approximately 19 mm tall and 9 mm wide.[7] In the transverse plane, the pedicles are oriented in the anterior-to-posterior plane and their angle increases from L1 to L5 (Fig. 2-2).[8] The L5 pedicles possess a posterolateral orientation[1] and have an elliptical shape, with the long axis rotated away from the vertical inferiorly. The pedicle sagittal angle (formed between the

12   A.O. Ortiz and H. Deramond

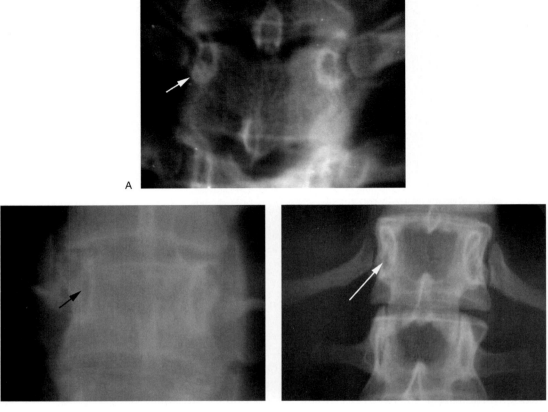

Figure 2-5. Thoracic vertebral bodies. AP views show relatively small pedicles (arrow) in the upper thoracic area (A), slight increase in the size (arrrow) in the midthoracic area (B), and relatively larger pedicles (arrow) at the thoracolumbar junction (C).

pedicle axis and the vertebral body equator) decreases from L1 to L5.[8] Therefore, although large, the pedicle orientation must be taken into account when transpedicular instrumentation is used.[9]

The thoracic pedicles are short and thin; they arise from the superior portion of the vertebral body and are directed dorsally and slightly cranially. They are well visualized at the superolateral portions of the vertebral bodies in frontal projection. The pedicle height and width tend to decrease from T1 to T4 and to increase gradually from T4 to T12.[10] The average pedicle heights and widths at T4, T8, and T12 are 10.4 and 3.7 mm, 11.2 and 4.8 mm, and 15.2 and 8.7 mm, respectively.[10] The thoracic pedicle length increases between T1 and T10 and then decreases slightly to T12, and the pedicle transverse angle decreases from T1 to T12.[10] This angle changes from 30° to 40° at T1 and T2 (Fig. 2-6), to 20° to 25° at T3 to T11; it measures 10° at T12.[1] A consistent

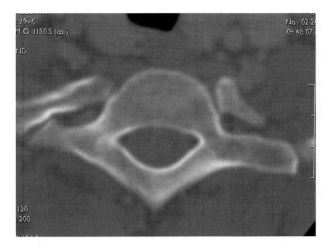

Figure 2-6. This axial CT scan shows the obliquity of the T1 pedicle.

trend or change has not been observed with respect to the thoracic pedicle sagittal angle. In the thoracic spine, the medial pedicle wall lies in close proximity to the thoracic spinal cord and the inferior and superior pedicle margins are located within 2 to 4 mm of the spinal nerve root (Fig. 2-7). The dura mater is closely

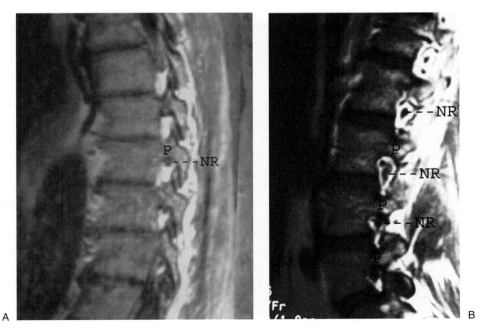

Figure 2-7. Proximity of the thoracic nerve root (NR) to the pedicle (P). (A) T1-weighted sagittal MR image at the level of the thoracic spine showing the intervertebral foramina. (B) T1-weighted sagittal MR image at the level of the lumbar spine showing prominent intervertebral foramina.

apposed to the pedicular margins of the thoracic spine.[11] In patients with thoracic pedicle screw placement, nerve root violation, nerve root compression, and cerebrospinal fluid leak are reported complications. These complications could theoretically occur during improper PV needle placement as a result of poor needle angulation, incorrect entry site, or insufficient pedicle size. To minimize the chance of a neurological complication in the thoracic spine, the operating physician must understand that the thoracic pedicle is uniquely different from the lumbar pedicle with respect to size and angulation. For the smallest thoracic pedicles (T3-T6), a small-diameter (13-gauge) needle or a parapedicular route should be used.

Cervical pedicles are characteristically small and form the posteromedial margin of the foramen transversarium that protects the vertebral artery. Because of their small size and proximity to the vertebral artery, spinal cord, and exiting nerve roots, the cervical pedicles are not suited for a transpedicular needle approach.

Vascular Anatomy

The arterial supply to the spine is segmental, and related to structures such as the vertebrae and paraspinal muscles, which derive from each somite. In the thoracic and lumbar spine, sacral, lumbar, and intercostal arteries provide the arterial supply to the vertebral column and its contents. The artery of the lumbar enlargement, also termed the artery of Adamkiewicz, originates from the T9-T12 intercostal arteries in 75% of cases and is more common on the left side.[12] This artery anastomoses with the anterior spinal artery and contributes blood supply to the anterior spinal cord. Damage to this important artery can theoretically occur from percutaneous instrumentation procedures, but it has not been reported in association with PV.

A basic understanding of the spinal venous system is helpful as an aid to recognizing cement leaks during PV. Three interconnecting valveless venous networks (interosseous, epidural, and paravertebral) make up the vertebral venous system. The trabecular compartment within the vertebral body contains numerous vascular channels, which can follow one or more drainage routes. These intramedullary venous channels can connect to the basivertebral plexus, which emerges from the posterior surface of the vertebral body, in the midline, and drains into the ventral epidural (internal vertebral) venous plexus. Alternatively, the vertebral body veins can course anteriorly and drain into the an-

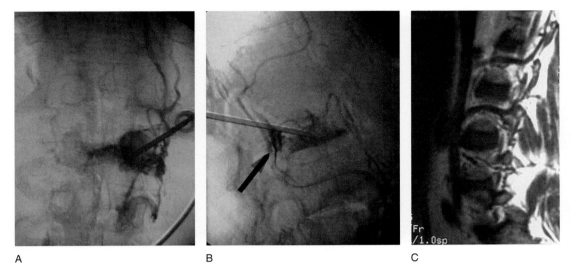

A   B   C

Figure 2-8. Venous drainage. (A) AP venogram of contrast injected into a vertebral body, showing a dense vertebral stain and a prominent ascending lumbar vein. (B) Lateral view obtained during the same injection showing the ventral epidural venous plexus (arrow). (C) T1-weighted sagittal MR image showing several large lumbar veins draining directly into the inferior vena cava.

terior external vertebral plexus, or course laterally and drain into the ascending lumbar or intercostal veins.

The basivertebral vein drains to the retrovertebral epidural venous plexus, a lattice of transverse and vertical venous channels directly behind the vertebral bodies. The ventral epidural venous plexus connects segmentally with the paravertebral plexus via the transversely oriented suprapedicular and infrapedicular veins. The paravertebral veins are largely vertical channels represented as follows: in the lumbar spine, by the ascending lumbar veins; in the thoracic spine, by the azygos and hemiazygos veins; and in the cervical spine, by the vertebral veins. Lumbar veins can drain into the inferior vena cava, the ascending lumbar vein, or the azygos vein (Fig. 2-8). The ascending lumbar vein drains into the azygos vein, iliac vein, or left renal vein. In the thoracic spine, the intercostal veins drain into the azygos (right side) or hemiazygos (left side) system, with ultimate drainage into the superior vena cava (Fig. 2-9). The vertebral veins join the subclavian veins just medial to the internal jugular veins. The venous connectivity between the very vascular vertebral body and both the epidural venous plexus and the inferior vena cava affords a direct route for cement embolization into the vascular system and the lungs during PV.

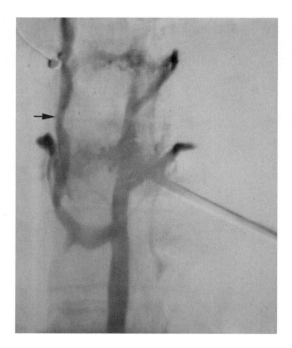

Figure 2-9. AP thoracic venogram showing the azygos vein (arrow).

To avoid the interosseous veins when the needle is inserted into the lateral part of the vertebral body, the tip of the needle should be placed into either the superior or inferior part of the vertebral body, not into the equatorial plane.

Paraspinal Soft Tissues

The deep muscles of the back are the posterior paraspinal structures. At the level of lumbar spine, the deep back muscles that directly attach to the spine include the erector spinae muscles and the multifidus muscles. During a percutaneous transpedicular approach, the needle goes through these deep muscles and reaches the posterior neural arch, where they attach directly to the spine. The risk of hemorrhage after bony puncture is very low because of the spontaneous compression by the muscle fibers. The parapedicular route is more risky because of the fatty components just outside the pedicle (Fig. 2-10): blood leakage could occur through the hole of the external part of the pedicle in a free space (retroperitoneal or extrapleural). The lateral needle position also precludes direct pressure to provide hemostasis (which can be easily applied after a transpedicular approach).

When performing PV, the operating physician must be aware

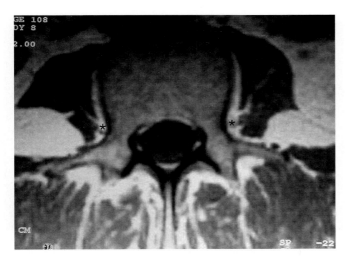

Figure 2-10. Fatty parapedicular tissue (asterisk) communicating largely with the retroperitoneal space.

that the anterior paraspinal soft-tissue structures vary with the level of the procedure and the site of needle insertion. In the lumbar spine, these structures include the liver, spleen, kidneys, adrenal glands, psoas muscle, aorta, and inferior vena cava. In the thoracic spine, the lung and aorta are in close proximity to the vertebral column. Caution is advised when approaching the thoracolumbar junction because the posterior costophrenic sulcus extends down to this level.

Percutaneous Approaches

Cervical Spine

In the cervical spine, the percutaneous approach is usually anterolateral. Because of the fatty environment of the jugulocarotid vessels, these structures are mobile and may be punctured during needle insertion. The vertebral arteries are fixed in a bony canal and must be avoided during needle introduction. A lateral approach should be avoided because of the risk to the vertebral arteries. Anatomical landmarks and structures differ according to the vertebral level.

Upper Cervical Level (C1-C2)
The approach for the upper cervical level is anterolateral and submandibular. The entry point of the needle is located just under the angle of the mandibula, and the route must avoid the submandibular gland, the jugulocarotid vessels, and the oropha-

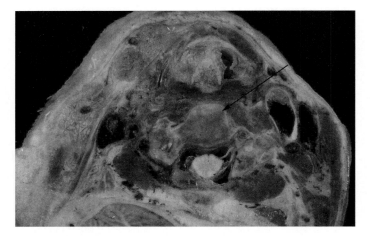

Figure 2-11. Axial anatomical view at the C1-C2 level (arrow, vertebral body).

ryngeal structures (Fig. 2-11). The C2 vertebral body is punctured from its inferior and lateral part (Fig. 2-12).

A report published in 2000 described a transoral approach that allowed access to C2. Because the posterior wall of the oropharynx is in proximity to C2, this approach does not put critical anatomical structures at risk for puncture or injury.[14] Nevertheless, for sterility reasons, the anterolateral approach is preferable.

Middle and Inferior Cervical Levels (C3-C7)
The approach to the middle and inferior cervical levels is anterolateral. The needle must avoid the thyroid gland.[15] It is pos-

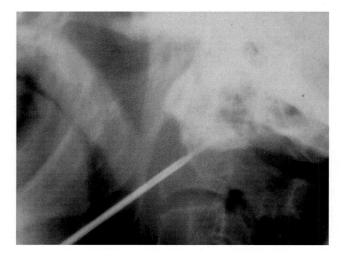

Figure 2-12. Lateral view showing the percutaneous approach to C2.

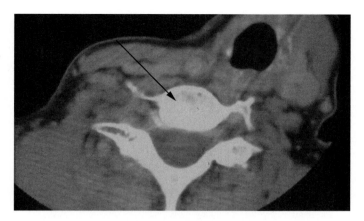

Figure 2-13. Axial CT view showing manually displaced tracheo-esophageal tract (arrow, vertebral body).

sible to pass medial or external to the jugulocarotid vessels. Tracheoesophageal tract and jugulocarotid vessels can be pushed away medially by finger pressure (Fig. 2-13), and the needle can be inserted just external to the vessels. These anatomical landmarks must be visualized on the preprocedure CT scan or during needle insertion (if CT guidance is used).

Thoracic Spine

In the thoracic spine, approaches of the vertebral body vary according to the vertebral thoracic level.

Upper Thoracic Level (T1-T3)

The upper thoracic level can be reached either by an anterolateral or posterolateral approach. The anterolateral approach is suprasternal and must avoid the different supraaortic vessels, the tracheoesophageal tract, and the thyroid gland (often in a cervicothoracic position) (Fig. 2-14). That approach must be visualized on a preprocedural CT scan. Most of the time, a right anterolateral approach is better, to avoid the esophagus. The anterolateral approach can be performed under a biplane or a C-arm fluoroscopy unit,[16] but the combination of CT scan with C-arm fluoroscopy is suggested. The transpedicular approach is preferred for safety reasons; in most cases, the pedicles of the upper thoracic spine can accommodate 13- or 15-gauge needles.

Middle and Lower Thoracic Levels (T4-T12)

Two posterolateral approaches can be used at the middle and lower thoracic levels: the transpedicular approach and the parapedicular approach above the transverse process.

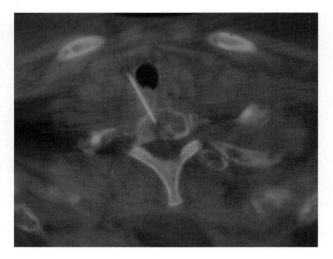

Figure 2-14. Axial CT scan showing suprasternal approach to T1-T2.

The transpedicular approach is the recommended approach for PV. The size of the needle must be adapted to the size of the pedicle. If the pedicle is too small, a parapedicular approach can be used.

The parapedicular approach, described as a CT-guided technique,[3] can be performed safely using a biplane or C-arm fluoroscopy unit. The initial trajectory is intercostal, and the needle is obliquely directed above the transverse process into the channel, limited externally by the posterior part of the rib and medially by the superior articular facet of the adjacent vertebra and the pedicle (Figs. 2-3 and 2-15). The route is protected from the pleura by the rib and from the spinal canal by the superior articular facet and pedicle.

The intercostal approach (Craig's technique) must be avoided for PV because the trajectory is just lateral to the neural foramina, which would put the nerves and vessels running into it at risk for injury.

Lumbar Spine

In the lumbar spine, percutaneous approaches are posterolateral transpedicular or parapedicular. According to the obliquity and size of the pedicles, the transpedicular route is used almost exclusively at the L5 level. The transpedicular route is preferred whenever possible because of its safety. The parapedicular approach above the transverse process is an acceptable alternative because it is located away from the important anatomical structures (kidneys, liver, spleen, spinal canal, neural foramina); the

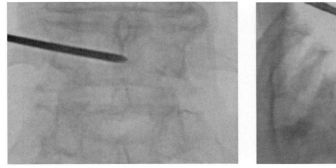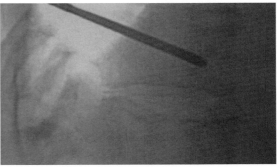

A   B

Figure 2-15. Parapedicular approach: AP (A) and lateral (B) views.

needle slides over the transverse process, along the lateral part of the superior articular facet, and then over the superolateral part of the pedicle to enter the bone at the anterior and lateral part of the pedicle (Fig. 2-16). When that approach is used, it is possible to insert the needle into the medial and anterior part of the vertebral body (Fig. 2-17). Craig's technique must also be

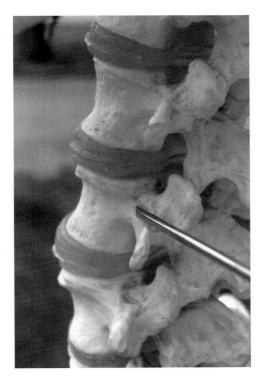

Figure 2-16. Model of the spine showing needle penetration in the lumbar region using the parapedicular approach.

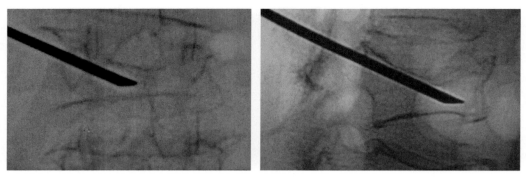

A

B

Figure 2-17. Lumbar parapedicular approach: AP (A) and lateral (B) views.

avoided for PV because the trajectory is just lateral to the neural foramina, which would put the nerves and vessels running into it at risk for injury.

References

1. Christenson PC. The radiologic study of the normal spine: cervical, thoracic, lumbar, and sacral. *Radiol Clin North Am* 1977; 15(2):133–154.
2. Gehweiler JA, Jr, Osborne RL, Jr, Becker RF. Osteology. In: *The Radiology of Vertebral Trauma.* Philadelphia: WB Saunders Co; 1980: 3–70.
3. Brugieres P, Gaston A, Heran F, et al. Percutaneous biopsies of the thoracic spine under CT guidance: transcostovertebral approach. *J Comput Assist Tomogr* 1990; 14(3):446–448.
4. Kothe R, O'Holleran JD, Liu W, et al. Internal architecture of the thoracic pedicle. An anatomic study. *Spine* 1996; 21(3):264–270.
5. Misenhimer GR, Peek RD, Wiltse LL, et al. Anatomic analysis of pedicle cortical and cancellous diameter as related to screw size. *Spine* 1989; 14(4):367–372.
6. Phillips JH, Kling TF, Cohen MD. The radiographic anatomy of the thoracic pedicle. *Spine* 1994; 19(4):446–449.
7. Panjabi MM, Goel V, Oxland T, et al. Human lumbar vertebrae. Quantitative three-dimensional anatomy. *Spine* 1992; 17(3):299–306.
8. Ebraheim NA, Rollins JR, Xu R, et al. Projection of the lumbar pedicle and its morphometric analysis. *Spine* 1996; 21(11):1296–1300.
9. Robertson PA, Stewart NR. The radiologic anatomy of the lumbar and lumbosacral pedicles. *Spine* 2000; 25(6):709–715.
10. Ebraheim NA, Xu R, Ahmad M, et al. Projection of the thoracic pedicle and its morphometric analysis. *Spine* 1997; 22(3):233–238.
11. Ebraheim NA, Jabaly G, Xu R, et al. Anatomic relations of the thoracic pedicle to the adjacent neural structures. *Spine* 1997; 22(14): 1553–1556.
12. Lasjaunias P, Berenstein A. *Surgical Neuroangiography.* New York: Springer-Verlag, 1990.

13. Craig FS. Vertebral-body biopsy. *J Bone Joint Surg* 1956; 38A(1):93–102.

14. Tong FC, Cloft HJ, Joseph GJ, et al. Transoral approach to cervical vertebroplasty for multiple myeloma. *Am J Roentgenol* 2000; 175(5): 1322–1324.

15. Brugieres P, Gaston A, Voisin MC, et al. CT-guided percutaneous biopsy of the cervical spine: a series of 12 cases. *Neuroradiology* 1992; 34(4):358–360.

16. Dufresne AC, Brunet E, Sola-Martinez MT, et al. [Percutaneous vertebroplasty of the cervico-thoracic junction using an anterior route. Technique and results. Report of nine cases.] *J Neuroradiol* 1998; 25(2):123–128.

3

Osteoporosis: Medical and Surgical Options

Abraham M. Obuchowski, Aleksandar Curcin, and John P. Kostuik

Osteoporosis is a common bone disease affecting nearly 200 million individuals worldwide. In the United States alone, there are more than 1.5 million osteoporotic fractures annually, including 250,000 hip, 250,000 wrist, and 500,000 to 700,000 vertebral fractures.[1] Although vertebral fractures are much more common, hip fractures are the most devastating, with a 12 to 20% mortality rate in the first 4 to 6 months after fracture.[2] Up to 25% of patients with hip fractures require long-term nursing care, and only one third of patients with hip fractures return to prefracture activity levels. Current estimates indicate that 10 million Americans already have the disease and an additional 18 million have osteopenia, putting them at risk of developing the disease. Of this at-risk population, 80% are women. However, 30% of hip fractures and 20% of vertebral fractures occur in men.[1]

In 1995 it was estimated that direct medical expenses for osteoporotic fractures exceeded $13.8 billion, accounting for 432,000 hospital admissions, an estimated 2.5 million physician visits, and 180,000 nursing home admissions in the United States.[3] With the increasing proportion of elderly in the population, costs are projected to rise to an estimated $130 billion in 2050.[4] Therefore, the institution of effective therapies for patients with or at risk for osteoporosis is of great importance in reducing the number of total osteoporosis-related fractures.

Osteoporosis is a skeletal disorder "characterized by low bone mass and microarchitectural deterioration of bone tissue, leading to increased bone fragility and a resultant increase in fracture risk."[5] Previously, osteoporosis was not diagnosed until a fracture occurred with signs of skeletal demineralization. Today, with the advent of bone density measurement techniques, osteoporosis can be diagnosed much earlier. Based on the World Health Organization's definition of osteoporosis, diagnosis is made by measuring bone mineral density (BMD).[6,7] Early diagnosis and current treatment options can reduce the incidence of fractures and their complications.

Decreased bone density or bone mass can occur because of failure to achieve optimal peak bone mass, bone loss secondary to increased resorption, or inadequate replacement of lost bone due to decreased bone formation. An individual's BMD is related to his or her peak bone mass at maturity. Peak bone mass is usually reached after puberty and continues into the third decade of life. Bone is remodeled throughout life, and bone mass remains stable for years after peak bone mass is reached, because the rate of bone resorption and bone formation are equal. As age increases, however, the rate at which bone remodeling occurs also increases, and the rate of bone resorption exceeds the rate of bone formation, resulting in a net loss of bone, or osteoporosis.

Loss of bone mass is therefore an integral part of aging that occurs in both men and women at an average rate of 0.6 to 1.2% per year from midlife on.[2,8] In women, menopause accelerates the rate of bone loss for the subsequent 5 to 8 years, with an annual loss of approximately 2 to 3% of trabecular bone and 1 to 2% of cortical bone. After 50 years of age, there is an exponential increase in the rate of fractures: one third of women will experience a vertebral fracture secondary to osteoporosis by age 65, and one out of every two white women will experience an osteoporotic fracture at some point in her lifetime. After maturity, women lose about 50% of their trabecular bone and 30% of their cortical bone mass. Men lose approximately two thirds of these amounts.[2]

Calcium and vitamin D are associated with the osteoporotic process. Calcium requirements rise at menopause owing to increased obligatory calcium loss and decreased gastrointestinal absorption, which persists throughout life. Vitamin D deficiency is important because age-related vitamin D deficiency causes calcium malabsorption, accelerated bone loss, and an increased fracture risk.

Despite all our attention to diet, exercise, and other modifiable lifestyle risk factors, genetic predisposition is by far the single most important factor in determining who will develop osteoporosis. For example, one study of twins suggested that 80% of the variation in peak bone mass can be attributed to genetically determined factors,[9] and another study found that a maternal history of hip fracture was associated with a twofold increased

Table 3-1 Risk Factors for Osteoporotic Fracture

Primary	Ankylosing spondylitis
Nonmodifiable	Chronic obstructive pulmonary disease
Personal history of fracture as adult	Cushing's syndrome
History of fracture in first-degree relative	Endometriosis
Caucasian race	Gastrectomy
Advanced age	Gonadal insufficiency
Dementia	Hyperparathyroidism
Woman	Hypophosphatasia
	Insulin-dependent diabetes mellitis
Potentially modifiable	Lymphoma, leukemia
Estrogen deficiency:	Malabsorption syndromes (Crohn's disease,
Early menopause (age < 45) or bilateral	celiac sprue)
oophorectomy	Multiple myeloma
Prolonged premenopausal amenorrhea	Rheumatoid arthritis
(> 1 yr)	Sarcoidosis
Smoking	Severe liver disease
Steroids	Thyrotoxicosis
Diet: poor intake or diseases causing	Tumor secretion of parathryroid hormone
decreased gastrointestinal absorption	
Low calcium intake	**Other**
Vitamin D deficiency	Anticonvulsants
Sedentary lifestyle	Cigarette smoking
Low body weight	Cytotoxic drugs
Poor health, frailty	Excessive alcohol
Recurrent falls	Excessive thyroxine
Impaired eyesight despite adequate	Glucocorticoids
correction	Gonadotropin-releasing hormone agents
	Heparin
Secondary	Lithium
Acromegaly	Tamoxifen (premenopausal use)
Addison's disease	

risk of hip fracture.[10] In addition, different alleles of the gene for vitamin D receptor may be associated with differences in bone mass and remodeling rates.[11,12] Although hormonal, dietary, and physical inactivity have only approximately a 20% influence in predicting or affecting one's risk of developing osteoporosis, educating patients about the importance of behavior and lifestyle modification to maintain healthy bone can alter several of the risk factors (Table 3-1).

Evaluation

Bone Mineral Density

Clinical evaluation of osteoporotic metabolic bone diseases includes bone densitometry and measurements of biochemical markers for bone resorption and bone formation. Dual-energy x-ray absorptiometry (DEXA) is commonly used to measure bone density,[13] but other methods include quantitative computerized tomography (QCT),[14] single- and dual-photon absorptiometry (SPA and DPA), and ultrasound.[15]

Single- and Dual-Photon Absorptiometry

Single-photon absorptiometry is limited to the appendicular skeleton, whereas DPA, which was developed to overcome this limitation, can be used to measure the density of the axial skeleton. Although the scans are easily performed, both methods use an isotope that decays with time, which necessitates complicated calibration corrections and quality control procedures. Reproducibility and precision are not as accurate as that with DEXA.[8] Furthermore, the bone density measurements obtained when SPA is used on the appendicular skeleton do not correlate well with vertebral body BMD and thus cannot substitute for direct vertebral density measurements.[8]

Dual-Energy X-Ray Absorptiometry

Dual-Energy x-ray absorptiometry has largely replaced the older SPA and DPA techniques because it is more accurate and provides reproducible values for bone mineral content and Bone mineral density in the lumbar spine, proximal femur, distal radius, and the entire body. Bone mineral density is calculated from the bone mineral content and the area of bone scanned (g/cm^2).

Dual-Energy x-ray absorptiometry offers several advantages: it is a safe procedure, with minimal radiation exposure (< 10 mrem); it has a short scanning time (approximately 3–5 min); it has a low incidence of reproducibility errors and variability of repeat readings (0.5–1.5%), facilitating the detection of small changes over time; and by allowing lateral patient positioning, which also provides an accurate measurement of the central trabecular portion of the vertebral body, it can avoid the falsely elevated readings of a standard AP radiograph secondary to osteophytes and aortic calcifications.

Quantitative Computed Tomography

Available in most radiology departments, QCT can evaluate true bone density (mg/cm^3), and it is the only method that can measure cancellous and cortical bone densities separately on a given bone; it can measure bone density in the axial, as well as in the appendicular, skeleton. Compared with DEXA, QCT's radiation exposure (100–300 mrem vs 10 mrem) is much greater, its precision and accuracy are lower (although still at acceptable levels), and its cost is much higher.[13]

Ultrasound

Ultrasound, particularly of the calcaneus (which is easily accessible), provides information on the underlying microarchitecture of bone and may predict fracture risk.[13] Ultrasound technology allows the measurement of the speed of sound and broadband ultrasound attenuation; speed of sound indicates bone density and elasticity, and broadband ultrasound attenuation reflects bone density as well as bone structure and composition.

Understanding Bone Densitometry Results

Bone mass or BMD values vary depending on the method (DEXA, SPA, DPA, or QCT) used to obtain them. Therefore, to standardize results, an individual's relative BMD is expressed in standard deviations from either the age-matched reference group or the young adult reference group. These relative values are known as the Z-score and T-score, respectively. For example, a T-score of −2 means that the patient's BMD is 2 standard deviations below the mean BMD for the young adult reference group.

According to the World Health Organization,[16] osteopenia is defined as a BMD between 1 and 2.5 standard deviations below the mean BMD of the young adult reference group, and osteoporosis is defined as a BMD 2.5 standard deviations or more below the mean BMD of the young adult reference group.

Clinical Examination

There is no general agreement about who should be screened or when screening should be performed. Based on the guidelines of the Scientific Advisory Board of the National Osteoporosis Foundation,[17] BMD screening is useful in menopausal women in whom BMD results may affect the decision to start hormone replacement therapy. Screening is recommended for (1) patients using estrogen therapy or an alternative therapy to protect the skeleton, such as estrogen-deficient women at risk for low bone density, (2) documenting reduced BMD in a patient with a radiographically documented vertebral abnormality or osteopenia, (3) diagnosing low bone mass in a patient taking steroids, (4) documenting low bone density in a patient with asymptomatic primary or secondary hypoparathyroidism, and (5) monitoring the efficacy of a therapeutic intervention for osteoporosis. Nevertheless, most patients are not diagnosed until after the first fracture, and the screening of normal premenopausal women is not effective.[18]

Whether osteoporosis is diagnosed on BMD screening or discovered after a fragility fracture, the workup should be the same. The history should include evaluation of calcium intake and diet, level of physical activity, smoking and alcohol history, menstrual and reproductive history, family history of osteoporosis, and history of other metabolic or endocrine disorders that might affect the skeleton. Minimal laboratory screening should include serum calcium, as an ionized calcium and fasting calcium excretion (easily measured as the calcium/creatinine ratio in the second-voided morning specimen).

Although most patients with fractures present with severe and debilitating pain, the clinician should be alert to the fact that sometimes vertebral fractures are clinically silent (i.e., not painful). Complications of vertebral compression fractures (VCFs) include chronic back pain, height loss, and exaggerated kyphosis.

Vertebral compression fractures can have a catastrophic effect on a patient's life: they can severely limit levels of activity, cause pain on standing or walking, make reaching for or holding an object (such as a milk container) difficult, and prevent normal bending. Multiple fractures in certain anatomical areas have additional potential consequences: in the thoracic area, they may cause restrictive lung disease, and in the lumbar area they may alter abdominal anatomy and cause constipation, abdominal distention, pain, and premature satiety with decreased appetite. Older patients with multiple fractures may become homebound and unable to shop or care for themselves. This new dependency and its alteration in lifestyle, superimposed on the chronic pain, which can strain relationships with spouse, family, and friends, often leads to what can be the most debilitating and overwhelming complication of all, depression.

Medical Treatment

Indications

A patient with a *T*-score lower than −2.5 on a standard DEXA scan, indicative of osteoporosis, should be managed with medicopharmacological treatment to prevent fractures. A *T*-score between −1 and −2.5 is consistent with osteopenia and should cause one to consider medical treatment based on the patient's overall risk profile.

A Z-score lower than −2 (i.e., a BMD that is 2 standard deviations below the age-matched reference group) indicates accelerated bone loss, and one should investigate for secondary causes of osteoporosis. Additionally, the workup should assess for secondary causes of bone mineral loss and should include measurements of phosphate, thyroid-stimulating hormone, 25-hydroxyvitamin D, complete blood count, and liver function; in some cases, parathyroid levels should be measured as well.

Interventions

The goal of therapy is to prevent fractures. A combination of exercise, vitamin and mineral supplements, and pharmacological agents is used.

Exercise

It is generally accepted that exercise and physical activity strengthen bones and muscles, improve balance and mobility, and decrease the risk of falling. Yet although a prospective co-hort study published in 1998[19] showed a dose–response rela-tionship between physical activity and hip fracture (the risk of hip fracture was reduced by 42% in the most intensely active women), the investigators found no such relationship between activity and vertebral or wrist fractures.

Pharmacological Agents, Vitamins, and Minerals

The process of bone resorption followed by synthesis of bone ma-trix and mineralization is known as coupling, and it may take up to 8 months per cycle. At any point in time, some bone will have been resorbed and not yet replaced. This unreplaced bone is referred to as the remodeling space. The remodeling space is in-creased in postmenopausal women. Most of the pharmacologi-cal agents used to treat osteoporosis (termed "referred anti-resorptive agents") result in a decrease in the remodeling space.

Estrogen replacement therapy has been the mainstay of phar-macological therapy because estrogen inhibits bone resorption, results in a small increase in bone density, decreases the risk of fracture, and decreases cardiovascular disease by approximately 50%. The cardiovascular effect is an important benefit because cardiovascular disease is the leading cause of death in post-menopausal women. Therefore, in the absence of contraindica-tions, estrogen has been the first drug of choice in the preven-tion and treatment of osteoporosis. One study suggested a possible 51% decrease in hip fracture and 27% risk reduction of other fractures.[20] However, the Food and Drug Administration (FDA) has withdrawn approval of estrogen as a treatment for os-teoporosis because of insufficient supporting data. Currently, es-trogen continues to be approved for the prevention of osteo-porosis. Many preparations exist, including oral and transdermal estrogens; the choice is based on tolerance and convenience. The most important contraindication to the use of estrogen is breast cancer or a strong family history of breast cancer. Relative con-traindications include gallbladder disease, thromboembolic dis-ease, and migraine headaches. The most common side effects are breast tenderness and return of menstrual bleeding. Other side effects include mood swings and gallbladder disease.

An amino bisphosphonate is a stable analogue of pyrophos-phate that attaches to the hydroxyapatite binding sites on both osteoblasts and osteoclasts. However, the binding affinity for these sites is four times more avid for osteoclast than for osteo-blast sites; 80% of the activity affects osteoclastic resorption. The net effect is to decrease bone resorption with an ultimate increase in bone density. Modification of the side chains of the bisphos-phonates results in the development of various compounds with different potencies to inhibit bone resorption. Gastrointestinal ab-sorption of this class of drugs is less than 10%.

Calcium intake, recommended for prevention and treatment of osteoporosis, ranges between 1 and 2 g/day. Most studies indicate that calcium decreases bone loss, but does not stop it. However, calcium supplementation alone has been associated with a decrease in new vertebral fractures.[21] There is no advantage to any particular formulation. In a study of 3270 institutionalized women in France treated with calcium (1200 mg/day) and vitamin D (800 IU/day) for 3 years,[22] investigators found a 43% decrease in hip fracture. In another study of women more than 60 years old whose diet contained less than 1000 mg of calcium per day, a calcium supplement of 1200 mg/day for a period of 4 years prevented bone loss at the forearm. There was a 59% reduction in vertebral fractures.[23]

Calcitonin inhibits the action of osteoclasts, thereby inhibiting bone resorption and resulting in increased BMD, particularly in patients with high bone turnover.[24] Calcitonin also has an analgesic effect on fracture pain and is therefore useful in the management of acute VCFs. Its mode of analgesic action is not known.

Selective estrogen receptor modulators comprise a new class of medications developed for the treatment of breast cancer and osteoporosis; these agents provide the beneficial effects of estrogen without its potential disadvantages. They bind to estrogen receptors and have estrogen-agonist effects on bone, lipids, and blood clotting as well as estrogen-antagonistic effects on the breast and uterus. A multicenter, randomized trial showed that treatment with selective estrogen receptor modulators was associated with a 30% reduction in VCF incidence in postmenopausal women with osteoporosis with or without previous fractures.[25]

Intervention Evaluation

For patients treated with estrogen, calcitonin, or selective receptor modulators, follow-up BMD testing is recommended every 2 to 4 years to evaluate efficacy. For patients treated with bisphosphonates, BMD testing is recommended at 1- to 2-year intervals.

Biochemical markers make it possible to analyze changes in bone formation and absorption. Osteocalcin, a noncollagenous matrix protein in bone, is produced exclusively by osteoblasts and is a marker for bone formation. Because normally there is a tight coupling of resorption and formation, osteocalcin also reflects bone turnover. Other markers for bone formation include alkaline phosphatase and procollagen peptides. Indicators of bone resorption include hydroxyproline, calcium and collagen cross-links, urinary pyridinium collagen cross-links, and cross-linked N-telopeptides or C-telopeptides for type I collagen. Urinary pyridinoline cross-link measurements correlate with histomorphometric assessments of bone turnover and resorption. These bone markers have been used in evaluating efficacy of treatment.

Surgical Treatment

The surgical treatment of osteoporotic VCFs begins with a correct diagnosis, determining whether the spine is stable or unstable. Stable VCFs usually are amenable to nonsurgical treatment, whereas unstable VCFs usually require surgery.

Diagnosis

Fracture Classification
In simplest terms, a VCF is a fracture in which the vertebral body partially collapses. Figure 3-1 shows the four types of VCFs as classified by Denis.[26] A fracture involving the superior end plate (type B) is the most commonly encountered VCF. Vertebral compression fractures typically present with involvement of the an-

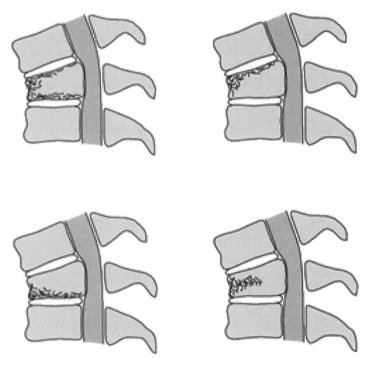

Figure 3-1. Four types of VCF as described by Denis. (From Denis, Ref. 26.)

terior vertebral cortex; however, some VCFs may involve the lateral cortex. The most important radiographic hallmark of these fractures is that the posterior vertebral body cortex (the medial column) is not compromised or disrupted.

Fracture Biomechanics

Several different force vectors (Fig. 3-2) can cause VCFs. The intrinsic alignment of the spine (kyphosis or lordosis) also has a direct influence on what type of fracture will result from a given loading scenario. Axial loads on the spine typically result in burst-type fractures in the cervical and lumbar spine because those regions are normally in lordosis, whereas in the thoracic spine (which has normal kyphosis), axial loads result in VCFs. When VCFs occur in the lumbar and cervical regions, they are caused by flexion. The resulting kyphosis increases the anterior bending moment on the thoracic region, placing that region at additional risk for VCFs.

Fractures in Weakened Bone

In patients with healthy bone stock, VCFs typically result from a substantial force that imparts considerable energy to the spine. Fractures of these types are seen in falls from a moderate height, skiing accidents, or relatively minor vehicular trauma. With appropriate treatment, these fractures rarely collapse to a greater extent than that seen on immediate postinjury radiographs. In patients with compromised bone density (e.g., those with osteoporosis), minor trauma (e.g., sitting down hard on a chair) or even activities of daily living (e.g., bending over to make a bed) often result in a VCF. Radiographs of these fractures obtained in

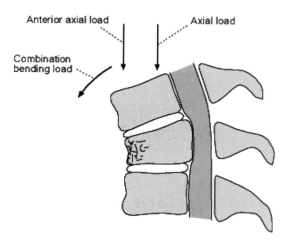

Figure 3-2. Force vectors contributing to VCF.

the immediate postinjury period may reveal a minor amount of collapse in the involved vertebra. However, these fractures, unlike those in patients with healthy bone stock, often continue to collapse.[27]

Stability

Determining Spinal Instability

For any patient with a spinal injury, a critical question in evaluation and treatment is whether the spine is "stable." Clinical *instability* of the spine has been defined as "the loss of the ability of the spine under physiological loads to maintain its pattern of displacement so that there is no initial or additional neurological deficit, no major deformity, and no incapacitating pain."[28] Those authors also described detailed systems for assessing spinal instability. Although an extensive discussion of such assessment is beyond the scope of this text, the reader is encouraged to become familiar with the details and application of White and Panjabi's criteria.[28]

Quick Assessment of Spinal Instability

Although precise definitions and criteria for spinal instability have been described, it is often helpful in daily clinical practice to be able to refer to quick "rules of thumb" in assessing a thoracic or thoracolumbar compression fracture for instability. The four essential parameters to consider are anterior collapse, segmental kyphosis, adjacent fractures, and weakening of posterior restraints. Anterior collapse is assessed by using the uninjured vertebrae above and below the fracture as guidelines for normal height comparison. If a fractured vertebra has more than 50% loss of height or collapse of the anterior vertebral cortex, relative to the height of the adjacent vertebrae, it should be considered to be potentially unstable.[29] Segmental kyphosis should be measured to include the fractured segment. For example, the segmental kyphosis in an L1 superior end plate fracture would be measured from the superior end plate of T12 to the inferior end plate of L1. If segmental kyphosis measures more than 25°, the fracture should be considered to be potentially unstable. Multiple adjacent fractures may have a greater impact on spinal stability than would result from an isolated fracture. Multiple adjacent fractures, whether all acute or a combination of adjacent acute and old fractures, should be scrutinized carefully and considered to be potentially unstable. A fracture that is suspected of having weakened the posterior column restraints (e.g., one that has stretched the posterior ligaments or facet joints), should be considered to be potentially unstable. The presence of more than two of these indicators of potential instability should serve as the impetus to apply more stringent criteria for instability, to follow the patient closely with serial examinations and radiographs, and to seek early subspecialist consultation.

Successive Fracture and Progressive Deformity

In the uninjured stable spine, there is a balance of forces acting about the spinal column's axis of rotation. In Figure 3-3, the lever arm z (uninjured spine) is acted upon by the weight of the body and is counteracted by the posterior column restraints acting at a lever arm $3z$. Note the relative increase in the anterior lever arm once a VCF has developed. At this point, there is relatively less force counteracting the anterior collapse of the spinal column. In patients with osteoporotic bone, the fracture continues to collapse, which increases the anterior lever arm even more, complicating the situation. As a result of the increased anterior lever arm, less force is required to produce subsequent fractures and a progressive kyphotic deformity.

Indications for Surgical Treatment

For patients with osteoporotic VCFs, *absolute* indications for surgical treatment include spinal cord or cauda equina compression with neurological deficit, progressive deformity (kyphosis or scoliosis) leading to pulmonary compromise, and progressive spinal deformity resulting in an imbalance of the trunk and torso. Patients with any one of these indications are counseled that surgical intervention is necessary to correct and reverse the damage caused by the fracture. *Relative* indications for surgical treatment

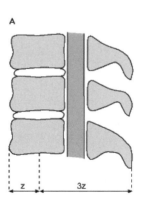
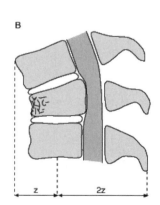
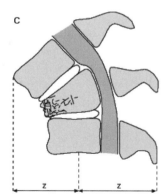

Figure 3-3. Biomechanical loading of the spine. (A) The lever arm z (uninjured spine) is acted upon by the weight of the body and is counteracted by the posterior column restraints acting at a lever arm $3z$. (B) Once a VCF has developed, there is a relative increase in the anterior lever arm, which results in relatively less force counteracting the anterior collapse of the spinal column. (C) In patients with osteoporotic bone, this situation is complicated by the fact that the fracture continues to collapse, which increases the anterior lever arm even more. As a result of the increased anterior lever arm, less force is required to produce subsequent fractures and a progressive kyphotic deformity.

include intractable pain and correction of spinal deformity for cosmesis. Patients in this category are advised that surgery may help alleviate their pain and correct an unsightly "hunchback" deformity.

Advantages of Surgical Treatment

The basic advantages of surgical treatment are the ability to decompress the spinal cord and nerves and to stabilize the spine rigidly with instrumentation. In patients with osteoporotic fractures and neural compression, a direct decompression procedure, such as a laminectomy, without adjunctive spinal instrumentation is rarely indicated. In formulating a surgical treatment plan, one must bear in mind that in the presence of a kyphotic deformity, the spinal cord and nerves are often compressed secondary to being "tented" across the apex of the deformity. In such cases, *indirect* decompression of the neural elements can often be achieved by restoring normal spinal alignment (Fig. 3-4). If spinal realignment and indirect decompression do not result in adequate relief of neural compromise then, in certain patients, more extensive direct decompression (vertebral corpectomy, laminectomy) may be necessary.

In some cases, surgical treatment with spinal instrumentation is performed solely to correct an existing deformity or halt a progressive deformity. In such an application, the instrumentation

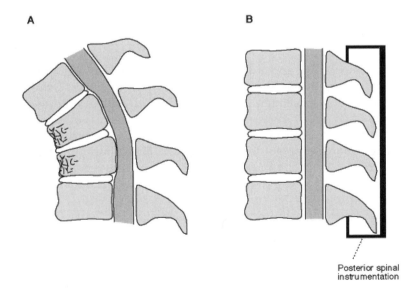

Figure 3-4. Indirect decompression achieved as a result of restoring spinal alignment.

acts as an internal splint for the spine. Typically, a posterior approach, with a combination of spinal rods, hooks, and/or screws, can result in substantial correction of deformity, prevention of further spinal collapse, and relief of pain. However, depending on the severity and rigidity of the deformity, surgical reconstruction may also require much more extensive combined anterior and posterior approaches to the spine.

Disadvantages of Surgical Treatment

Typically, patients with osteoporotic VCFs are elderly with substantial systemic comorbidities (e.g., cardiac disease, diabetes). As a result, surgical treatment can precipitate associated medical complications. Achieving stable fixation of the spinal implants can be problematic because of the underlying weakened bone. Accordingly, the spinal rods, hooks, and screws may become dislodged from the bone, resulting in loss of fixation and deformity correction. Once spinal instrumentation has been affixed to an injured segment of the spine, that portion of the spinal column becomes relatively stiffer than the adjacent segments. This alteration in the local biomechanics can place the adjacent vertebral bodies (typically the vertebra above the top of the instrumentation) at higher risk for subsequent VCFs. Some spine surgeons advocate intraoperative vertebroplasty in the adjacent segments to address proactively the potential for an adjacent segmental fracture (see sections entitled Indications, in Chapter 4, and Prophylactic Therapy, in Chapter 12). However, such intervention has not been conclusively documented as a proven benefit.

Summary/Conclusions

Patient morbidity and mortality are reduced when osteoporosis prevention regimens, including lifestyle modification and the use of pharmacological agents, are implemented. All patients should be educated about their risk factors and options for reducing the risk of fracture. They should also be informed about the value of regular exercise and adequate calcium and vitamin D intake. Treatment decisions should be based on each individual patient's medical history and personal preferences. Patients with unstable spines should not be considered for treatment with PV, and a subspecialty consultation should be obtained. When surgery is indicated, the clinician must keep in mind the problems of instrumentation fixation in the osteoporotic spine.

References

1. Riggs BL, Melton LJ, III. The worldwide problem of osteoporosis: insights afforded by epidemiology. *Bone* 1995; 17(5 suppl):505S–511S.

2. Riggs BL, Wahner HW, Dunn WL, et al. Differential changes in bone mineral density of the appendicular and axial skeleton with aging: relationship to spinal osteoporosis. *J Clin Invest* 1981; 67(2):328–335.

3. Ray NF, Chan JK, Thamer M, et al. Medical expenditures for the treatment of osteoporotic fractures in the United States in 1995: report from the National Osteoporosis Foundation. *J Bone Miner Res* 1997; 12(1):24–35.

4. Johnell O. The socioeconomic burden of fractures: today and in the 21st century. *Am J Med* 1997; 103(2A):20S–25S.

5. Consensus development conference: prophylaxis and treatment of osteoporosis. *Osteoporos Int* 1991; 1(2):114–117.

6. Consensus Development Conference: prophylaxis and treatment of osteoporosis. *Am J Med* 1991; 90(1):107–110.

7. Kanis JA, Melton LJ, III, Christiansen C, et al. The diagnosis of osteoporosis. *J Bone Miner Res* 1994; 9(8):1137–1141.

8. Riggs BL, Melton LJ, III. Involutional osteoporosis. *N Engl J Med* 1986; 314(26):1676–1686.

9. Young D, Hopper JL, Nowson CA, et al. Determinants of bone mass in 10- to 26-year-old females: a twin study. *J Bone Miner Res* 1995; 10(4):558–567.

10. Cummings SR, Nevitt MC, Browner WS, et al. Risk factors for hip fracture in white women. Study of Osteoporotic Fractures Research Group. *N Engl J Med* 1995; 332(12):767–773.

11. Eisman JA. Vitamin D receptor gene alleles and osteoporosis: an affirmative view [editorial]. *J Bone Miner Res* 1995; 10(9):1289–1293.

12. Tokita A, Kelly PJ, Nguyen TV, et al. Genetic influences on type I collagen synthesis and degradation: further evidence for genetic regulation of bone turnover. *J Clin Endocrinol Metab* 1994; 78(6):1461–1466.

13. Ryan PJ, Fogelman I. The bone scan: where are we now? *Semin Nucl Med* 1995; 25(2):76–91.

14. Engelke K, Grampp S, Gluer CC, et al. Significance of QCT bone mineral density and its standard deviation as parameters to evaluate osteoporosis. *J Comput Assist Tomogr* 1995; 19(1):111–116.

15. Bauer DC, Gluer CC, Genant HK, et al. Quantitative ultrasound and vertebral fracture in postmenopausal women. Fracture Intervention Trial Research Group. *J Bone Miner Res* 1995; 10(3):353–358.

16. Kanis JA, WHO Study Group. Assessment of fracture risk and its application to screening for postmenopausal osteoporosis: synopsis of a WHO report. *Osteoporosis Int* 1994; 4(6):368–381.

17. LeBoff MS. Metabolic bone disease. In: Kelley WN, Ruddy S, Harris ED, Jr, et al. eds. *Textbook of Rheumatology*. 5th ed. Philadelphia: WB Saunders Co; 1997:1563–1580.

18. Hayes WC, Piazza SJ, Zysset PK. Biomechanics of fracture risk prediction of the hip and spine by quantitative computed tomography. *Radiol Clin North Am* 1991; 29(1):1–18.

19. Gregg EW, Cauley JA, Seeley DG, et al. Physical activity and osteoporotic fracture risk in older women. Study of Osteoporotic Fractures Research Group. *Ann Intern Med* 1998; 129(2):81–88.

20. Hulley S, Grady D, Bush T, et al. Randomized trial of estrogen plus progestin for secondary prevention of coronary heart disease in

postmenopausal women. Heart and Estrogen/Progestin Replacement Study (HERS) Research Group. *JAMA* 1998; 280(7):605–613.

21. Reid IR, Ames RW, Evans MC, et al. Long-term effects of calcium supplementation on bone loss and fractures in postmenopausal women: a randomized controlled trial. *Am J Med* 1995; 98(4):331–355.

22. Chapuy MC, Arlot ME, Duboeuf F, et al. Vitamin D_3 and calcium to prevent hip fractures in the elderly women. *N Engl J Med* 1992; 327:1637–1642.

23. Recker RR, Hinders S, Davies KM, et al. Correcting calcium nutritional deficiency prevents spine fractures in elderly women. *J Bone Miner Res* 1996; 11(12):1961–1966.

24. Civitelli R, Gonnelli S, Zacchei F, et al. Bone turnover in postmenopausal osteoporosis. Effect of calcitonin treatment. *J Clin Invest* 1988; 82(4):1268–1274.

25. Ettinger B, Black DM, Mitlak BH, et al. Reduction of vertebral fracture risk in postmenopausal women with osteoporosis treated with raloxifene: results from a 3-year randomized clinical trial. Multiple Outcomes of Raloxifene Evaluation (MORE) Investigators. *JAMA* 1999; 282(7):637–645.

26. Denis F. The three column spine and its significance in the classification of acute thoracolumbar spinal injuries. *Spine* 1983; 8:817–831.

27. Lyritis GP, Mayasis B, Tsakalakos N, et al. The natural history of the osteoporotic vertebral fracture. *Clin Rheumatol* 1989; 8(suppl 2): 66–69.

28. White AA, Panjabi MM. *Clinical Biomechanics of the Spine.* 2nd ed. Philadelphia: JB Lippincott Co, 1990.

29. Garfin SR, Blair B, Eismont FJ, et al. Thoracic and upper lumbar spine injuries. In: Browner BD, Jupiter JB, Levine AM, et al. eds. *Skeletal Trauma: Fractures, Dislocations, Ligamentous Injuries.* 2nd ed. Philadelphia: WB Saunders Co; 1998:947–1034.

4

Patient Evaluation and Selection

M.J.B. Stallmeyer and Gregg H. Zoarski

Vertebral compression fractures (VCF) result from osteoporosis, malignant primary or metastatic bone tumors, and benign infiltrative tumors such as vertebral hemangiomas. Pain relief constitutes the primary indication for percutaneous vertebroplasty (PV). The effectiveness of PV for prophylaxis in the absence of local pain and tenderness remains unproven. In considering whether a patient may be a candidate for PV, it is important to use both clinical and imaging assessment. When patients are properly selected and evaluated, this procedure has provided substantial pain relief in 75 to 90% of patients with benign fractures[1-4] and in 59 to 86% of patients with malignant VCFs.[2,4-8]

Etiology

Osteoporosis

The most common cause of VCF is primary osteoporosis, also called "osteoporosis of aging." More than 700,000 symptomatic VCFs occur each year in the United States, and most of them occur in postmenopausal women.[9,10] The radiographic prevalence of thoracic or lumbar VCFs (defined as a loss of more than 15% of vertebral body height[10]) has been reported to be as high as 25% in a random sample of 85-year-old white women[11] and as high as 26% in women more than 50 years old. The radiographic incidence of VCF rises from 5/1000 women at age 50 to 54 years to nearly 30/1000 women at age 85 and older.[10]

Vertebral compression fractures have been associated with impairment of physical, functional, and psychosocial performance in older women.[12] Furthermore, the survival of patients who have had osteoporotic VCFs is lower, and this value diverges steadily from expected values. This difference increases with increasing duration of follow-up.[13]

Primary osteoporosis is characterized by decreased bone mass, with an associated increase in susceptibility to fractures, particularly in the axial skeleton, femur, and wrist. Most osteoporotic VCFs occur spontaneously (46%) or after only minimal trauma (36%), and a correct diagnosis at first visit to a health care provider is made in only 43% of the cases.[14] Chronic steroid use, which accelerates bony resorption by osteoclasts, predisposes patients to secondary osteoporosis and insufficiency fracture. This population includes patients taking steroids for asthma or chronic obstructive pulmonary disease, transplant patients, and some patients with malignancies such as multiple myeloma and lymphoma.

Patients with osteoporotic VCFs usually present with acute pain and tenderness over the spine at, or very near, the level of radiographic compression deformity. The fractures are located most frequently at the thoracolumbar junction and usually occur after minimal trauma, although they may be described as having occurred "spontaneously." Plain radiographs show diffuse osteoporosis and often reveal additional healed VCFs (Fig. 4-1). Although computed tomography (CT) is the best modality for determining whether the fracture line extends through the posterior wall of the vertebral body, such a finding is the exception rather than the rule in osteoporosis. Bone scintigraphy can help localize the symptomatic fracture and may aid in differentiating acute from chronic fractures. However, bone scans may show increased uptake for as long as 12 months after a fracture and should be interpreted with this fact in mind (Fig. 4-2). A positive bone scan at the level of a VCF has been shown to be highly predictive of a positive clinical response after PV. In one study, subjective pain relief was achieved in 26 of 28 (93%) PV procedures.[15] However, that study did not compare the predictive value of scintigraphy with magnetic resonance (MR) imaging.

Magnetic resonance images can show characteristic changes in marrow signal that depend on the age of the fracture.[16] Acute and subacute fractures, defined as fractures 2 to 30 days old, are hypointense in signal on T1-weighted images and hyperintense on T2-weighted and short tau inversion recovery (STIR) sequences (Fig. 4-3). Blood products, usually subacute, may occasionally be found along the end plates of the affected vertebra. After 30 days, most osteoporotic VCFs become isointense to normal bone on all three sequences (Fig. 4-4). Cuenod et al.[17] described a band of hyperintense T2 signals adjacent to the frac-

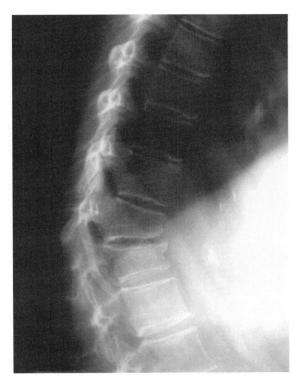

Figure 4-1. Lateral chest radiograph showing adjacent osteoporotic thoracolumbar VCFs that occurred when this patient lifted a bag of groceries.

tured end plate in 48 percent of benign VCFs. They also observed that these fractures became isointense to normal vertebrae after administration of gadolinium contrast.

In some cases of benign osteoporotic VCF, there may be retropulsion of a posterior bone fragment into the spinal canal, usually along the superior end plate (Fig. 4-4).[17] Radiculopathy is rare but has been reported.[18] Severe neurological deficit or spinal cord compression is even more unusual.[19] In Kümmell's disease, thought to be a result of avascular necrosis, a fluid collection forms along the superior end plate after osteoporotic collapse (Fig. 4-5).[20–22] The role of MR image in the preoperative evaluation of patients with osteoporotic VCFs and Kümmell's disease for PV was recently reviewed and summarized.[23]

Healed VCFs may show normal marrow signal or may appear hypointense on both T1- and T2-weighted sequences due to sclerosis. When suspected, sclerosis should be evaluated and confirmed by CT; injection of polymethylmethacrylate (PMMA) in such cases is typically impossible or yields suboptimal results with respect to pain reduction (Fig. 4-6).

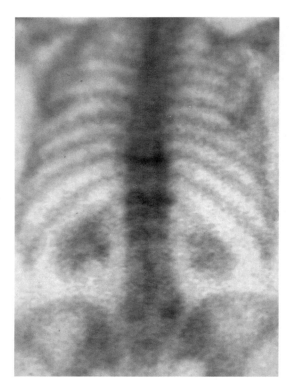

Figure 4-2. Radionuclide bone scan showing increased uptake at the levels of acute T10 and T12 osteoporotic VCFs.

Malignant Compression Fractures

Common causes of malignant VCFs include osteolytic metastases and multiple myeloma. The clinical history in patients with malignant VCFs is often straightforward and known to the physician. In some cases, however, distinguishing between benign and malignant causes of VCF can be problematic. In questionable cases, a biopsy performed coaxially through the PV needle can often provide a diagnosis at the time of intervention. Similar to patients with osteoporotic VCFs, patients with malignant VCFs usually present with acute pain and tenderness over the spine at or very near the level of radiographic deformity. Radiculopathy is not a contraindication to PV; however, patients should be warned about the possibility that PV will not relieve, or might even worsen, these symptoms. Symptomatic spinal cord compression at the level of the VCF is a clear contraindication to PV; injection of PMMA could worsen symptoms or could complicate corrective decompressive surgery. However, PV may be a reasonable consideration for the treatment of a painful VCF after the canal has been decompressed.

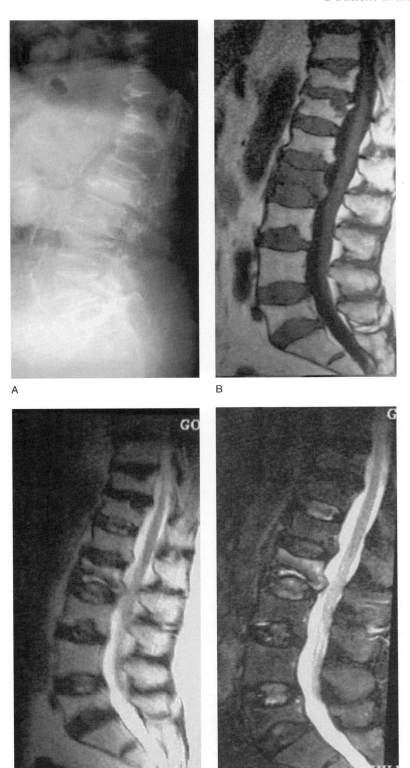

A

B

C

D

Figure 4-3. This patient with osteoporosis and multiple lower thoracic and lumbar vertebral compression deformities complained of focal pain and tenderness. (A) Lateral spine radiograph. (B) Sagittal T1-weighted MR image showing acute and chronic osteoporotic fractures. The acutely compressed L2 vertebra showed hypointense marrow signal. Other compressed vertebrae showed normal marrow signal, indicating old, healed fractures. (C) T2-weighted MR image showing heterogeneously increased signal in the L2 vertebral body, representing fracture edema. (D) Sagittal STIR MR image showing prominent hyperintense signal in L2 with characteristic localization to the upper portion of the vertebral body. On examination under fluoroscopy, L2 was the most painful level.

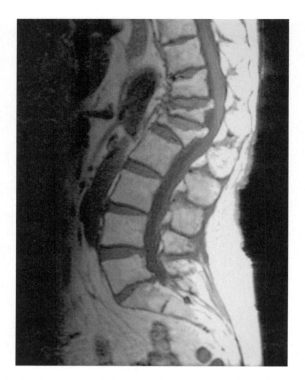

Figure 4-4. Sagittal T1-weighted MR image showing old osteoporotic fractures at T11, T12, and L1. Note retropulsion of posterior–superior margins of T12 and L1.

Most malignant bone lesions appear on plain radiographs as focal lytic lesions within the vertebral body, with destruction or focal rarefaction of bony trabeculae. Rarely, there may be expansion of the contours of the bone. A radionuclide bone scan may show increased uptake, but it may be normal or equivocal, particularly in patients with myeloma. Thin-section (≤ 3 mm) CT images through potentially malignant lesions may yield useful information about the integrity of the posterior wall of the vertebral body before PV is performed. In one study, at least partial destruction of the posterior vertebral body wall was reported in more than 50% of patients with malignant lesions who were treated with PV.[4]

Findings from MR studies that are suggestive of malignant VCF include heterogeneous marrow or bright enhancement, rather than the return to isointensity that is seen in benign osteoporotic VCFs after contrast injection. Short tau inversion recovery sequences, with fat suppression, are helpful in identifying VCF edema; heterogeneous or diffuse hyperintensity on STIR and T2-weighted sequences is typical of malignant disease (Fig. 4-7).[16]

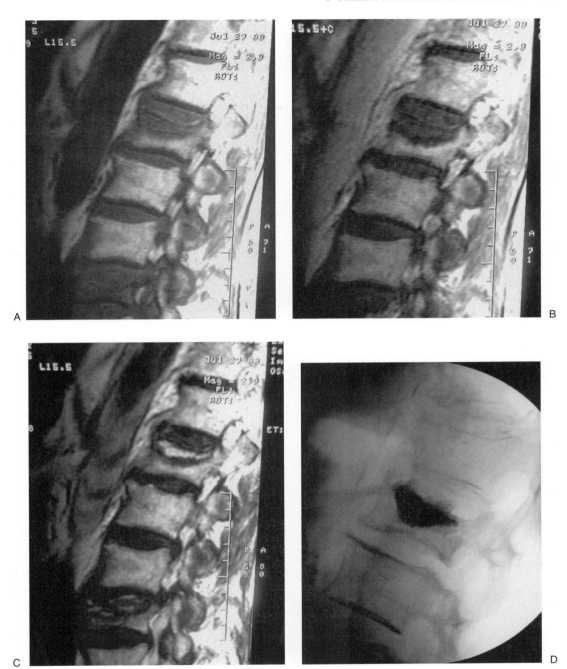

Figure 4-5. This 95-year-old woman had a painful L1 compression fracture. (A) T1-weighted MR image showing markedly diminished signal along the upper vertebral end plate. (B) Postcontrast T1-weighted MR image showing no enhancement in abnormal region of vertebra. (C) T2-weighted MR image showing compression fracture of L1 with fluid along superior end plate and subjacent sclerotic bone. Avascular necrosis (Kümmell's disease). (D) Lateral image after PV showing deposition of cement in the region of avascular necrosis and fluid accumulation. The patient reported substantial pain relief.

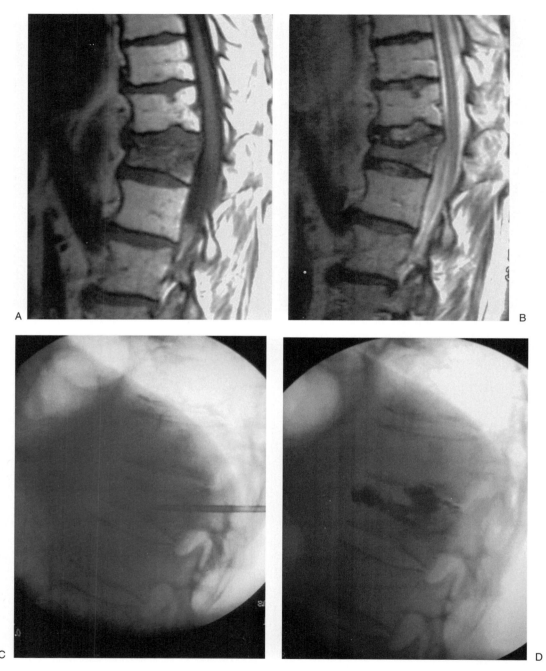

Figure 4-6. This 68-year-old man had long-standing thoracolumbar compression fracture and back pain. Sagittal T1-weighted (A) and T2-weighted (B) MR images showing hypointense signal in the fractured T12 vertebral body, indicating sclerosis rather than edema. (C) Lateral view showing increased density of T12 compared with neighboring vertebral bodies. Placement of needles for cement injection was very difficult because of increased bone density. (D) Lateral view after PV, showing relatively little intraosseous deposition of cement and minor extrusion into the disk space.

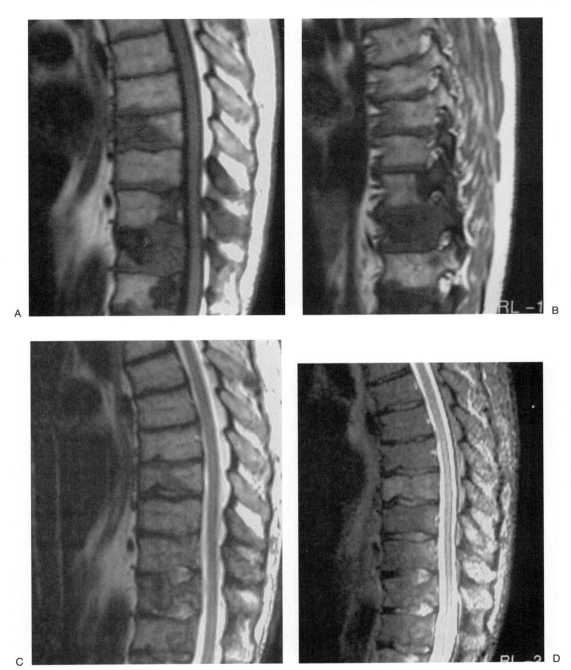

Figure 4-7. This 51-year-old man had metastatic adenocarcinoma. (A) Sagittal T1-weighted MR image showing multiple hypointense foci of marrow replacement within lower thoracic vertebrae. (B) T1-weighted MR image showing foci of malignant marrow replacement within multiple pedicles. (C) T2-weighted MR image showing intermediate but heterogeneous signal throughout the vertebral bodies. (D) Sagittal STIR MR image showing increased signal intensity within metastatic foci. The more homogeneous high signal represented edema from a partial pathological compression fracture of a midthoracic vertebra.

Reports that hypointensity or isointensity to adjacent vertebrae on diffusion-weighted sequences was indicative of malignancy[24] were refuted in 2000.[25]

Diffuse malignant spinal involvement is seen more often in hematopoietic malignancies than with metastases.[26] Other findings suggestive of malignant vertebral invasion include abnormal signal in the posterior elements (seen more often in metastases than in myeloma), bony expansion (convex posterior cortex of a vertebra, or expansion of the contour of the posterior elements), and an epidural soft-tissue mass.[16,17] In some patients, however, imaging findings remain equivocal, and biopsy before or at the time of PV may provide the only definitive answer (Fig. 4-8).

In patients with multiple myeloma, distinguishing between benign VCFs caused by secondary osteoporosis or steroid treatment and diffuse myelomatous skeletal involvement can be difficult. The distribution of lesions in myeloma is often strikingly similar to that seen in benign osteoporotic fractures. Upper thoracic involvement, however, may favor a diagnosis of myeloma.[27]

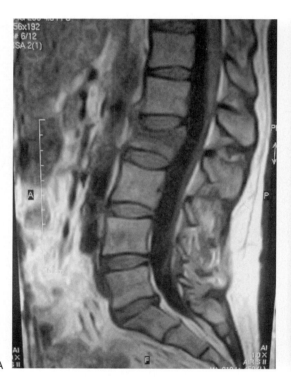
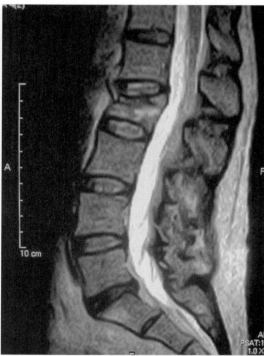

A   B

Figure 4-8. Traumatic VCF. (A) Sagittal T1-weighted MR image 6 weeks after a motor vehicle collision, showing hypointensity and compression of L2. Posterior expansion suggested the possibility of metastatic disease. (B) T2-weighted MR image showing hyperintense signal at the level of the VCF. Multiple biopsies showed no malignancy.

Vertebral Hemangiomas

Vertebral hemangiomas (VH) are common benign lesions of the spine, found in 5 to 11% of autopsies.[28] Most VHs occur as single lesions. Usually, they are asymptomatic and discovered only incidentally during radiographic examination. Rarely, VHs may cause pain with or without the presence of a pathological VCF. Asymptomatic as well as symptomatic lesions are more likely to be located in the thoracic region.[29,30] Some VHs may exhibit aggressive characteristics, including marked expansion of the contours of the vertebral body and extension of the tumor outside the vertebra with nerve root or spinal cord compression.[29,31,32]

Plain radiographs may reveal a coarse, exaggerated, vertically striated trabecular pattern within the vertebral body, sometimes extending into pedicles or bulging the posterior cortical margin (Fig. 4-9A). Thin-section (≤ 3 mm) CT evaluation is usually worthwhile for evaluating the integrity of the posterior wall of the vertebral body or the posterior encroachment upon the spinal canal (Fig. 4-9B).

Imaging of VHs by means of MR techniques typically shows a circumscribed, mottled lesion that is hyperintense compared with normal bone marrow on both T1- and T2-weighted sequences.[33] The mottled MR image appearance and signal are consistent with the histological finding of adipose tissue and thickened bony trabeculae. Alternatively, more active VHs may appear hypointense on MR image sequences when vascular channels predominate (Fig. 4-9C).[30] In such cases, VHs typically enhance more densely than normal bone marrow (Fig. 4-9D). Injection of PMMA or *n*-butyl cyanoacrylate has been performed for analgesia or control of operative blood loss in patients with spinal VHs; posterior bulging into the epidural space is commonly reported and is not a contraindication to PV.[34] Although PV is generally contraindicated for a patient with spinal cord compression, preoperative PMMA injection has been reported to consolidate the vertebral body and to reduce the risk of massive hemorrhage associated with decompressive laminectomy and resection of epidural VHs.[35]

Patient Selection

Appropriate patient selection is essential to achieving clinical success with PV. More than 80% of the population will suffer from back pain at some point in life.[36,37] Thus, patients with etiologies of back pain such as spinal stenosis or disk disease may be encountered more frequently than patients with appropriate

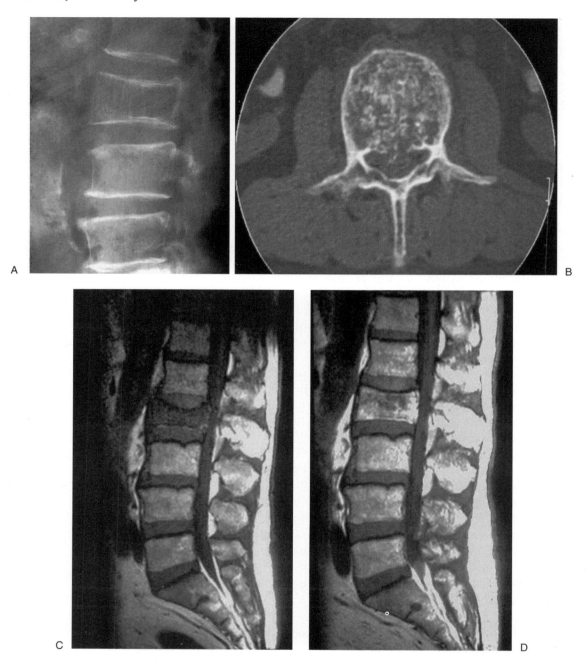

Figure 4-9. This patient had focal back pain and tenderness. (A) Lateral radiograph showing coarse vertical trabecular striations characteristic of VH. (B) Axial CT through L2 confirmed trabecular thickening typical of VH. Expansion of posterior cortex resulted in narrowing of the spinal canal. (C) Sagittal T1-weighted MR image showing deformity and hypointense signal within L2. (D) Postcontrast T1-weighted MR image showing enhancement of L2 VH. Again, note expansion of posterior cortical margin.

indications for treatment with PV. Physicians practicing PV will need an efficient screening mechanism to avoid being overwhelmed by requests to see inappropriate patients and to review their radiographs for possible PV.

Indications

The primary indication for performing PV is pain associated with a VCF caused by osteoporosis, VH, lytic infiltration, or tumor invasion. Treatment for painful tumor infiltration without fracture also seems reasonable, but few data exist to evaluate the efficacy of PV for this particular indication. It is not clear whether PV should be performed before radiation therapy or reserved for patients who have already received maximal doses of therapeutic radiation. In our experience, PV does not diminish the effects of radiation therapy given after the PMMA injection. Irradiation has not been shown to alter the cured PMMA.[38]

Prophylactic PV may play a role in the future for patients at extremely high risk for VCF (e.g., patients with severe and symptomatic kyphosis due to previous osteoporotic VCFs, patients taking chronic steroid treatment who have sentinel pain). Prophylaxis, however, is not yet an accepted indication for PV, and no studies have been undertaken to substantiate the efficacy of performing PV for prophylaxis.

The best clinical success is generally achieved in patients with pain and tenderness on palpation that is localized to the level of radiographic VCF. In early treatment series, most patients had unsuccessfully undergone conventional medical therapy consisting of analgesics and bed rest before PV was performed.[3] More recent series have advocated treatment as early as a few weeks[1] after the acute onset of a painful VCF that requires parenteral narcotics and hospitalization. Many operating physicians now treat such patients during the first week after fracture. Late treatment (> 6 months) is less likely to be successful in relieving pain, but numerous investigators have anecdotally reported symptomatic improvement with PV performed even years after the initial injury.

Younger patients with normal bone mineral density (BMD) and traumatic VCFs are not usually considered candidates for PV. However, PV has been appropriately and successfully used for patients less than 50 years old with other vertebral conditions. For example, it eliminated pain and the need for narcotic analgesics secondary to multiple-steroid-induced VCFs in a 36-year-old woman with systemic lupus erythematosus,[39] and it resulted in rapid pain relief in a 25-year-old man with collapse of L2 due to previously irradiated Langerhans cell histiocytosis.[40]

Contraindications

Emergent performance of PV is rarely, if ever, required. Osteo-myelitis or epidural abscess are absolute contraindications to PV with PMMA. In addition, coagulopathy must be corrected before the placement of a large-bore bone needle, and the procedure should be postponed in patients with fever or sepsis until they are afebrile.

Fractures with more than 70% loss of vertebral height are technically difficult to treat. Even with precise needle trajectory, the operating physician may find it difficult (or impossible) to achieve satisfactory needle placement within the remaining vertebral body height. In 2000, however, both a diminished need for analgesics (5/6) and reduced pain (5/6) were documented in six patients with more than 65 to 70% compression of low thoracic or lumbar vertebrae treated with bipedicular PV.[41] By positioning the bone needles in the lateral aspect of the vertebral bodies, the operating physicians were able to inject an average of 5.2 mL of opacified PMMA. There were no clinical complications. Despite these encouraging results, there seems to be little or no benefit in attempting to treat a true vertebra plana.

Traumatic VCFs in young, otherwise healthy patients should not be treated with PV until the long-term effects of PMMA injection have been studied and described. Symptomatic relief can be obtained in most cases with oral analgesics and bracing. Such patients, who are presumed to possess normal osseous restorative capability, generally heal their fractures and experience a substantial decrease in pain within 4 to 6 weeks.

Although radiculopathy is not a contraindication to PV, patients should be warned about the possibility that these symptoms may not be successfully treated (or in some cases may be worsened) with PV. As previously noted, malignant spinal cord compression or substantial spinal stenosis at the level of the compressed vertebra is at the very least an important relative contraindication to PV.

Although the posterior vertebral wall is usually intact in the case of osteoporotic VCF, this may not be the case with malignant lesions. The integrity of the posterior vertebral wall should be evaluated with CT before PV for malignant lesions because, if it is destroyed by tumor, there may be an increased risk of ventral epidural extravasation of cement. In addition, the risk of complications is higher for treatment of vertebral conditions associated with malignant lesions than for those associated with osteoporosis.[1–4,8,42]

Response to Requests from Patients and Physicians

Standard response letters to referring physicians and self-referred patients are helpful in screening patients for PV. Response letters should contain a discussion of the appropriate indications for the procedure, how the procedure is performed, and instructions on how to initiate the consultation process with either a primary care physician or the physician performing the PV. Other strategies for facilitating efficient screening, and for marketing a practice, could include patient and physician brochures, or incorporation of this information in a web page (e.g., spinefracture.com).

Screening of the Physician-Referred Patient

An appropriate clinical history, physical examination, and relevant radiographic studies should be obtained as the first step in evaluation of the PV candidate. This information helps differentiate the pain of VCF from that of other etiologies such as disk herniation, spinal cord or nerve root compression, discogenic back pain, facet arthropathy, or spinal stenosis.

Clinical history obtained from the referring physician should include a discussion of the precipitating event leading to VCF. In general, VCF pain is described by the patient as occurring acutely, usually after minimal trauma. Pain generally worsens with weight bearing and is often at least partially relieved by recumbency. Physical examination by the referring physician should demonstrate pain and tenderness corresponding closely to the level of fracture deformity. In the presence of multiple levels of compression, successful identification of the target level can often be accomplished only after thoughtful analysis of physical examination results combined with studies such as MR imaging or bone scans.

It is important to determine whether the etiology of a VCF might be due to underlying malignancy. A referring physician's office notes aid considerably in deciding well in advance whether a biopsy should be performed before cement injection.

Screening of the Self-Referred Patient

Initial evaluation of the self-referred patient is often considerably more difficult because this population tends to include not only patients for whom PV may be indicated but also patients with other causes of chronic back pain. It is important to stress that PV will not improve disease processes such as disk herniation, spinal stenosis, or facet and sacroiliac joint arthropathy.

Ideally, the patient should be referred to his or her primary care physician to undergo a focused history and physical examination. The primary care physician may also be a necessary component in the process of obtaining insurance approval for additional imaging that may be needed before the procedure, referral for preprocedure consultation, or approval for the PV procedure itself.

Preprocedure Consultation

Once imaging and clinical findings have been reviewed, and it has been determined that the patient may be an appropriate candidate for PV, a preprocedure consultation with the patient and interested family members may be arranged. Meeting with the family members involved in the patient's care is particularly important in the case of elderly or debilitated patients. Alternatively, and for patients who must travel a long distance for treatment, consultation can be performed on the day of the procedure.

It is helpful to begin by reviewing the history and clinical findings with the patient. Important points to discuss include the history of the fracture, including the time of onset of symptoms, precipitating factors such as trauma, the premorbid status of the patient, the patient's expectations, the impact on activities of daily living, and analgesic use. It is also helpful to know whether previous similar episodes of pain have occurred, and if so, how they resolved. A brief clinical examination can help identify the approximate location of pain and tenderness for correlation with imaging findings. This examination will also serve as an opportunity to evaluate the patient's overall condition and readiness to undergo PV, potential difficulties of prone patient positioning, contraindicated medications such as anticoagulants, and unique sedation requirements.

Most patients and families will be somewhat familiar with PV through popular press and Internet articles. The consultation should nevertheless include a brief discussion of how the procedure is performed at the specific institution, as well as detailed instructions about the ingestion of medications on the day of the procedure, diet instructions, what to expect during the procedure, and information on postprocedure care, transport to home or a health care facility, and the expected course of recovery. The preprocedure consultation is also a time to discuss potential treatment complications. If the procedure is performed by a trained operating physician (with adequate fluoroscopic imaging and appropriate opacification of cement), serious clinical complications should be extremely rare. The most commonly encountered complication is localized pain and tenderness at the needle sites in the first 72 h after the procedure, usually due to local bruising; this will resolve with mild analgesics such as ibuprofen or acetaminophen (see Chapter 10 for details).

To enhance the safety of injection and increase opacity, sterile barium sulfate, tungsten, or tantalum has been added to PMMA preparations. With these additions, however, the cement injected is no longer the same medical device approved by the Food and Drug Administration (FDA). The operating physician should address this fact with the patient at the time of consultation.

It is important to consider patient and family expectations during the consultation. If the patient is a good candidate for PV and the fracture is subacute, a good response can be expected: 80 to 90% of patients report substantial pain relief. However, if the fracture has been present for many months or years, there is a diminished likelihood of a clear clinical success. If a patient has multiple symptomatic VCFs, staging options should focus on treating the most painful VCFs first, or choosing target levels that may help prevent additional kyphotic deformity. A thorough discussion of staging strategy may also prevent disappointment, should the patient's pain not be substantially alleviated during the first treatment session.

Patient Instructions and Procedures

Instructions

For PV procedures performed during the morning, the patient should not ingest anything (except for medications) after midnight. If the procedure is scheduled for the afternoon, the patient should not ingest anything for at least 4 h before the scheduled time to permit safe administration of medication for conscious sedation.

In general, patients are advised to take their usual medications with sips of water on the day of the procedure. Diabetic patients scheduled for a morning procedure should be instructed to adjust their insulin dosage. Patients on anticoagulants should discontinue these medications at an appropriate interval before the procedure, but only after consultation with the primary care or prescribing physician.

Preprocedure Laboratory Studies

Routine examinations that should be obtained before PV include complete blood count, prothrombin time, activated partial thromboplastin time or international normalized ratio, activated clotting time, and platelets. If intraosseous venography is contemplated, laboratory evaluation of blood urea nitrogen and creatinine may also be ordered.

Examination under Fluoroscopy

Although in many cases it is possible to make a reasonable correlation between the general area of pain described by the patient and the level of VCF on radiographic studies, it is always a good idea to confirm this impression by examining the patient under fluoroscopy immediately before performing PV. This is especially true for patients with multilevel disease who report diffuse pain and tenderness and for those who may have difficulty precisely localizing discomfort.

Careful palpation over the posterior elements is performed to identify the most painful vertebral levels. With the patient prone, thumb pressure over each spinous process, or gentle side-to-side movement of a spinous process, often elicits tenderness in the presence of an acute VCF. Pressure and palpation over paravertebral muscles (i.e., parasagittal palpation) may also help identify whether muscle spasm constitutes an additional component of the patient's pain.

Summary/Conclusions

With careful review of clinical and imaging findings using the foregoing guidelines, identification of patients for whom PV is likely to have a successful outcome is often straightforward. Identification of patients unlikely to benefit can be time-consuming, but it is often equally straightforward. For physicians just beginning their PV practice, the ideal first patient is one with a single-level osteoporotic VCF, with focal pain well localized to the level of radiographic abnormality. With additional experience, more complex patients with multilevel fractures or fractures secondary to neoplasms can be treated as well.

References

1. Cyteval C, Sarrabere MP, Roux JO, et al. Acute osteoporotic vertebral collapse: open study on percutaneous injection of acrylic surgical cement in 20 patients. *Am J Roentgenol* 1999; 173(6):1685–1690.
2. Gangi A, Dietemann JL, Mortazavi R, et al. CT-guided interventional procedures for pain management in the lumbosacral spine. *Radiographics* 1998; 18(3):621–633.
3. Jensen ME, Evans AJ, Mathis JM, et al. Percutaneous polymethyl methacrylate vertebroplasty in the treatment of osteoporotic vertebral body compression fractures: technical aspects. *Am J Neuroradiol* 1997; 18(10):1897–1904.
4. Deramond H, Depriester C, Galibert P, et al. Percutaneous vertebroplasty with polymethyl methacrylate. Technique, indications, and results. *Radiol Clin North Am* 1998; 36(3):533–546.
5. Weill A, Chiras J, Simon JM, et al. Spinal metastases: indications for and results of percutaneous injection of acrylic surgical cement. *Radiology* 1996; 199(1):241–247.
6. Cortet B, Cotten A, Boutry N, et al. Percutaneous vertebroplasty in patients with osteolytic metastases or multiple myeloma [see comments]. *Rev Rhum Engl Ed* 1997; 64(3):177–183.
7. Cotten A, Dewatre F, Cortet B, et al. Percutaneous vertebroplasty for osteolytic metastases and myeloma: effects of the percentage of lesion filling and the leakage of methyl methacrylate at clinical follow-up. *Radiology* 1996; 200(2):525–530.

8. Kaemmerlen P, Thiesse P, Jonas P, et al. Percutaneous injection of orthopedic cement in metastatic vertebral lesions [letter]. *N Engl J Med* 1989; 321(2):121.

9. Melton LJ, III. How many women have osteoporosis now? *J Bone Miner Res* 1995; 10(2):175–177.

10. Melton LJ, III, Kan SH, Frye MA, et al. Epidemiology of vertebral fractures in women. *Am J Epidemiol* 1989; 129(5):1000–1011.

11. Johansson C, Mellstrom D, Rosengren K, et al. Prevalence of vertebral fractures in 85-year-olds. Radiographic examination of 462 subjects. *Acta Orthop Scand* 1993; 64(1):25–27.

12. Lyles KW, Gold DT, Shipp KM, et al. Association of osteoporotic vertebral compression fractures with impaired functional status. *Am J Med* 1993; 94(6):595–601.

13. Cooper C, Atkinson EJ, Jacobsen SJ, et al. Population-based study of survival after osteoporotic fractures. *Am J Epidemiol* 1993; 137(9): 1001–1005.

14. Patel U, Skingle S, Campbell GA, et al. Clinical profile of acute vertebral compression fractures in osteoporosis. *Br J Rheumatol* 1991; 30(6):418–421.

15. Maynard AS, Jensen ME, Schweickert PA, et al. Value of bone scan imaging in predicting pain relief from percutaneous vertebroplasty in osteoporotic vertebral fractures. *Am J Neuroradiol* 2000; 21(10): 1807–1812.

16. Baker LL, Goodman SB, Perkash I, et al. Benign versus pathologic compression fractures of vertebral bodies: assessment with conventional spin-echo, chemical-shift, and STIR MR imaging. *Radiology* 1990; 174(2):495–502.

17. Cuenod CA, Laredo JD, Chevret S, et al. Acute vertebral collapse due to osteoporosis or malignancy: appearance on unenhanced and gadolinium-enhanced MR images. *Radiology* 1996; 199(2):541–549.

18. Heggeness MH. Spine fracture with neurological deficit in osteoporosis. *Osteoporos Int* 1993; 3(4):215–221.

19. Salomon C, Chopin D, Benoist M. Spinal cord compression: an exceptional complication of spinal osteoporosis. *Spine* 1988; 13(2):222–224.

20. Kümmell H. Über die traumatischen Erkrankungen der Wirbelsaule. *Dtsch Med Wochenschr* 1895; 21:180–181.

21. Brower AC, Downey EF, Jr. Kummell disease: report of a case with serial radiographs. *Radiology* 1981; 141(2):363–364.

22. Dupuy DE, Palmer WE, Rosenthal DI. Vertebral fluid collection associated with vertebral collapse. *Am J Roentgenol* 1996; 167(6):1535–1538.

23. Do HM. Magnetic resonance imaging in the evaluation of patients for percutaneous vertebroplasty. *Top Magn Reson Imaging* 2000; 11(4): 235–244.

24. Baur A, Stabler A, Bruning R, et al. Diffusion-weighted MR imaging of bone marrow: differentiation of benign versus pathologic compression fractures [see comments]. *Radiology* 1998; 207(2):349–356.

25. Castillo M, Arbelaez A, Smith JK, et al. Diffusion-weighted MR imaging offers no advantage over routine noncontrast MR imaging in

the detection of vertebral metastases. *Am J Neuroradiol* 2000; 21(5): 948–953.

26. Kim HJ, Ryu KN, Choi WS, et al. Spinal involvement of hemato-poietic malignancies and metastasis: differentiation using MR imaging. *Clin Imaging* 1999; 23(2):125–133.

27. Lecouvet FE, Vande Berg BC, Maldague BE, et al. Vertebral compression fractures in multiple myeloma. Part I. Distribution and appearance at MR imaging [see comments]. *Radiology* 1997; 204(1): 195–199.

28. Schmorl G, Junghanns H. *The Human Spine in Health and Disease* (Besemann EF, transl. ed.). 2nd ed. New York: Grune & Stratton, 1971.

29. Krueger EG, Sobel GL, Weinstein C. Vertebral hemangioma with compression of spinal cord. *J Neurosurg* 1961; 18:331–338.

30. Laredo JD, Assouline E, Gelbert F, et al. Vertebral hemangiomas: fat content as a sign of aggressiveness. *Radiology* 1990; 177(2):467–472.

31. Ghormley RK, Adson AW. Hemangioma of vertebrae. *J Bone Joint Surg* 1941; 23(4):887–895.

32. McAlister VL, Kendall BE, Bull JWD. Symptomatic vertebral hemangiomas. *Brain* 1975; 98:71–84.

33. Ross JS, Masaryk TJ, Modic MT, et al. Vertebral hemangiomas: MR imaging. *Radiology* 1987; 165(1):165–169.

34. Cotten A, Deramond H, Cortet B, et al. Preoperative percutaneous injection of methyl methacrylate and *n*-butyl cyanoacrylate in vertebral hemangiomas. *Am J Neuroradiol* 1996; 17(1):137–142.

35. Ide C, Gangi A, Rimmelin A, et al. Vertebral haemangiomas with spinal cord compression: the place of preoperative percutaneous vertebroplasty with methyl methacrylate. *Neuroradiology* 1996; 38(6): 585–589.

36. Wells N. *Back Pain*. London: Office of Health Economics, 1985.

37. Roland MO, Morrell DC, Morris RW. Can general practitioners predict the outcome of episodes of back pain? *Br Med J (Clin Res Ed)* 1983; 286(6364):523–525.

38. Murray JA, Bruels MC, Lindberg RD. Irradiation of polymethyl methacrylate. In vitro gamma radiation effect. *J Bone Joint Surg* 1974; 56A(2):311–312.

39. Mathis JM, Petri M, Naff N. Percutaneous vertebroplasty treatment of steroid-induced osteoporotic compression fractures. *Arthritis Rheum* 1998; 41(1):171–175.

40. Cardon T, Hachulla E, Flipo RM, et al. Percutaneous vertebroplasty with acrylic cement in the treatment of a Langerhans cell vertebral histiocytosis. *Clin Rheumatol* 1994; 13(3):518–521.

41. O'Brien JP, Sims JT, Evans AJ. Vertebroplasty in patients with severe vertebral compression fractures: a technical report. *Am J Neuroradiol* 2000; 21(8):1555–1558.

42. Chiras J, Deramond H. Complications des vertebroplasties. In: Saillant G, Laville C, eds. *Echecs et Complications de la Chirurgie du Rachis. Chirurgie de Reprise*. Paris: Sauramps Medical; 1995:149–153.

Biomechanical Considerations

Stephen M. Belkoff

Percutaneous vertebroplasty (PV) has enjoyed rapid acceptance as a procedure to stabilize vertebral compression fractures (VCFs) and to prevent fractures in vertebral bodies weakened by osteolytic tumors. Although the procedure is being performed with increasing frequency, scientific investigations into basic questions regarding the clinical efficacy and technical aspects of the procedure are in their infancy. This chapter presents a review of the current body of knowledge regarding PV fundamental research, addresses PV-related issues (such as possible mechanisms for pain relief, biomechanical considerations regarding the stabilization of mechanically compromised vertebral bodies, the types of cement available, and the mechanical consequences of altering the composition of those cements) and relates results from recent basic research on PV to the clinical perspective.

Mechanism of Pain Relief

The augmentation and stabilization of vertebra using acrylic cement as an open procedure (vertebroplasty) has been practiced for many years.[1–10] However, the percutaneous introduction of cement into a vertebra was first reported in 1987.[11] The procedure consisted of injecting polymethylmethacrylate (PMMA) cement through a large-bore needle into a painful vertebral hemangioma (VH) that had aggressively consumed a C2 vertebra. The VH was injected primarily to prevent subsequent collapse of the involved vertebra, but the procedure also reportedly resulted in marked pain relief.[11] The procedure was quickly adapted to stabilize osteoporotic VCFs.[12] Since the introduction of PV, retrospective and prospective studies have reported pain relief in approximately 90% of patients treated for osteoporotic VCFs[13,14] and in 70% of patients treated for various tumors.[15,16] Although the exact mechanism of pain relief is unknown and may differ in patients with osteoporotic VCFs and those with tumors, possible mechanisms include thermal, chemical, and mechanical factors.[17,18]

Thermal

It has been hypothesized that the heat of polymerization causes thermal necrosis of neural tissue and is therefore the mechanism responsible for pain relief.[17] When PMMA polymerizes, heat is generated in the exothermic polymerization reaction.[19] Concern about potential thermal tissue injury caused by the heat of polymerization has been the topic of orthopedic investigations, with particular reference to arthroplasty.[19-22] Thermal injury illustrates an Arrhenius relationship in which temperature magnitude and exposure time are both critical factors. Thermal necrosis of osteoblasts occurs when temperatures are higher than 50°C for more than 1 min,[23,24] but apoptosis occurs when osteoblasts are exposed to lower temperatures for longer periods of time.[25] Some investigators have measured temperatures as high as 122°C during polymerization,[26] but the volumes of cement required to generate such temperatures are substantially greater than those typically used in PV.[26] Neural tissue may be more sensitive than osteoblasts to temperature.[27]

A recent ex vivo study suggests that temperature is not a mechanism of pain relief.[28] In that study, thermocouples were placed at three locations inside vertebral bodies (Fig. 5-1) to assess the

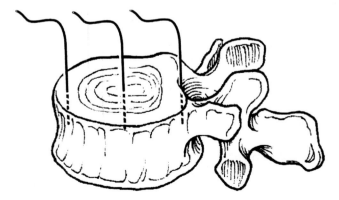

Figure 5-1. Schematic of a vertebral body instrumented with thermocouples to measure temperature elevation caused by polymerizing PMMA cement. Thermocouples were placed at the anterior cortex, at the centrum, and under the venus plexus of the spinal canal.

risk of thermal injury to interosseous nerves, periosteal nerves, and the spinal cord. The vertebral bodies received concurrent bipedicular injections totaling 10 mL of PMMA cement. Although temperatures exceeded 50°C for more than 1 min at the anterior cortex and in the center of the vertebral body, the authors concluded that temperature was an unlikely mechanism of pain relief for several reasons (Fig. 5-2). First, the experimental model did not include active heat transfer due to blood profusion, which would be expected to remove much of the heat in vivo. Second, 10 mL of injected cement is more than is typically used for PV.[29] And third, the cement was injected in a nonclinical fashion; that is, it was injected concurrently via both pedicles to maximize the thermal effect for experimental measurement. Typically, PV is performed as a staged procedure in which half the cement is first injected through one cannula placed in a pedicle.[18] Then the remaining cement is injected through the other cannula placed in the contralateral pedicle. The heat of polymerization from the initial injection would likely have partially dissipated before the second injection is made. For these reasons, it seems unlikely that temperature plays a role in pain relief.

Temperature may still play a role in slowing tumor growth.[21] A study published in 1999 indicated that apoptosis likely occurs in osteoblasts exposed to 48°C for 10 min or more.[25] If similar results are found for tumor cells, it will be possible to suggest that apoptosis and diminished tumor cell proliferation result from exposure to polymerizing PMMA.

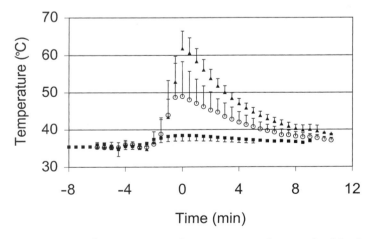

Figure 5-2. Typical temperature–time response of a vertebral body injected with 10 mL of PMMA cement. Temperatures of 50°C for more than 1 min cause necrosis of osteoblasts.

Chemical

Methylmethacrylate (MMA) monomer is cytotoxic,[30] but it is unknown whether concentrations present in vivo immediately after PV are high enough to be neurotoxic and therefore a mechanism of pain relief.[17] In vitro concentrations exceeding 10 mg/mL have been shown to be toxic to leukocytes and endothelial cells,[30] yet there are no reports that suggest in vivo concentrations reach such magnitudes. During knee arthroplasty, blood serum levels immediately after cementation and tourniquet release have been measured as high as 120 μg/mL, but such levels are typically much lower (< 2 μg/mL) and drop precipitously minutes after cementation.[31] Blood serum concentrations between 0.02 and 59 μg/mL have been measured during total hip replacement.[32] The volumes of cement used for hip and knee arthroplasty are two to three times greater than those typically used with PV, and the monomer concentrations measured for those procedures are 10 to 100 times less than MMA concentrations reported to be cytotoxic to tissue cultures.[30] Even though the cement used with PV is typically prepared with a greater monomer-to-polymer ratio than cement used for arthroplasty, it seems unlikely that MMA toxicity is responsible for pain relief experienced with PV.

Cytotoxicity has also been implicated in the autotumoral effect noted clinically.[33] However, a recent cell culture study[34] suggested that MMA monomer is cytotoxic to breast cancer cells in concentrations similar to those for leukocytes and endothelial cells.[30] Thus, it also seems unlikely that MMA monomer leachate from cement injected during PV has an antitumoral role. Nevertheless, until intravertebral MMA concentrations have been measured in vivo, the hypothetical cytotoxic effect of MMA monomer will remain in question.

Mechanical

Mechanical stabilization of the affected vertebral body appears to be the most likely mechanism of pain relief. As with fixation of fractures in other parts of the human skeleton, internal fixation (in the current case, by PV) likely stabilizes the fracture and prevents micromotion at the fracture site, thereby limiting painful nerve stimulation.[35,36] In tumors, the pain relief mechanism may be more complex. If the vertebral body contains regions of instability resulting from osteolytic activity by the tumor, PV may prevent micromotion and subsequent pain. If the cement injected during PV has some antitumoral effect,[33] then the pain associated with rapid tumor growth may be diminished. The antitumoral effect may be thermal or chemical, as mentioned earlier, but may also result from ischemia caused by the mechanical displacement of tumor tissue by the cement and resulting hydrostatic pressure. Thus, injecting PMMA cement into tumors of the spine may have the triumvirate effect of vertebral body stabilization, pain relief, and tumor growth impediment.

Biomechanical Stabilization

Basic Biomechanics

The spine serves to transmit loads from the upper body through the pelvis into the lower extremities. The spine is conceptually divided into three columns: anterior, medial, and posterior. The medial and anterior columns serve to resist axial compressive loads[37] that increase in magnitude from the cervical region to the lumbar region. Because the center of gravity of the human body is located anterior to the spinal column, it creates a combined load resulting in axial compression and an anterior bending moment. For the spine to remain erect, tensile forces along the posterior column (i.e., paraspinous muscles and ligaments) need to act about the medial column, which serves as a fulcrum, while the anterior column acts to resist compression (Fig. 5-3). During

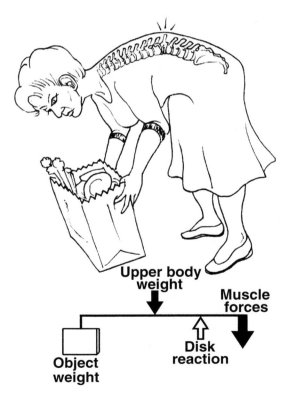

Figure 5-3. The body's center of gravity is anterior to the spine, creating an anterior bending moment and axial compression on the spine. Anterior flexion increases the anterior bending moment, thereby increasing the stresses on the spine and placing the spine at risk for fracture.

anterior flexion—for example, bending over to tie a pair of shoes—the body's center of gravity moves anteriorly, increasing the bending moment on the spine and the compressive stresses on the anterior column. Bending over to pick up a load not only moves the center of gravity anteriorly, but also increases the magnitude of the anteriorly located load, which, combined with the increased moment arm, dramatically increases the compressive stresses on the anterior column. It is this excessive compressive stress that results in VCFs. By definition, VCFs exhibit disruption of the anterior column.[37]

Compressive strength of vertebra is roughly related to the square of the vertebral bone mineral density (BMD).[38] When a patient's BMD is 2 standard deviations below the average for the sex-, height-, weight-, and race-matched young population, the patient is considered to be osteopenic. When BMD drops below 2.5 standard deviations, the patient is considered to be osteoporotic.[39] In patients with osteoporosis, vertebral BMD might be half what it was in their youth, which means the vertebral compressive strength may be as low as one fourth of what it was in their previous young healthy condition.

Although many VCFs go undiagnosed,[40,41] 700,000 VCFs are reported each year in the United States,[42] 300,000 to 400,000 of which result in hospital admissions. Vertebral compression fractures that are diagnosed may be immediately radiographically apparent or may present with pain but little or no radiographically discernible deformity.[43] The former fracture type is typically associated with an acute onset of pain (during lifting, raising a window, etc.), whereas the latter type suggests an initial weakening (perhaps as a result of microfractures) that reportedly progresses into radiographically diagnosable wedge fractures 6 to 16 weeks later.[43]

Volume Fill

The goals of stabilization for VCFs are similar to those of stabilization for fractures in other sites in the body, namely, to prevent painful micromotion and to provide a mechanically stable and biologically conducive environment for fracture healing to occur. The amount of strength and stability needed to provide the optimal mechanical environment for VCF healing is unknown. Early in the PV experience, complete injection of the anterior column of the vertebrae was thought to be necessary,[44] but recent clinical and experimental data have suggested that smaller volumes of cement may be sufficient. In one clinical study, 29 patients treated with PV received injected volumes ranging from 2.2 to 11.0 mL (mean, 7.1 mL) of cement; 90% of the patients experienced pain relief.[13] Barr et al.[45] indicated that injection of 2

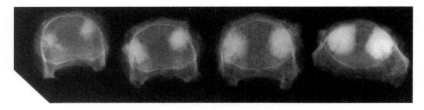

Figure 5-4. Radiograph of typical cement (Simplex P) distribution when 2, 4, 6, or 8 mL are injected into lumbar vertebrae.

to 3 mL into the thoracic and 3 to 5 mL into the lumbar regions resulted in 97% moderate to complete pain relief. These results suggest that pain relief may be achieved with smaller volumes, but no correlation of level treated, volume injected, and clinical outcome was explicitly reported. In osteolytic metastases and myeloma, there is reportedly no correlation between the percentage of lesion filled and pain relief.[29]

A recent ex vivo study attempted to determine the relationship between cement volume injected and subsequent mechanical stabilization and found that only 2 mL of PMMA was needed to restore strength in osteoporotic vertebral bodies (Fig. 5-4), but larger volumes (4–8 mL) were needed to restore stiffness.[46] The report suggested that stiffness is the mechanical parameter likely to be most closely linked with pain relief. Restoring initial strength would be expected to prevent refracture of the treated vertebra, whereas restoring initial vertebral body stiffness likely prevents micromotion and the pain associated with it. However, fully restoring prefracture stiffness to vertebral bodies may not be necessary or even desirable. As with other fractures, providing some mechanical stability, even less than that of the prefracture state, may be sufficient to allow healing.[47] If the repair is too stiff, stress shielding may occur and impede fracture healing. If the repair is not stiff enough, excessive motion at the fracture site may occur, resulting in nonunion. The volume and material properties of cement needed to achieve sufficient stabilization for healing and to prevent pain are yet unknown and can be definitively determined only by a prospective, controlled, randomized clinical study.

Unipedicular Injection

In another ex vivo study, Tohmeh et al.[36] found in that vertebral body strength may be restored via a unipedicular injection of 6 mL of cement without risk of vertebral body collapse on the uninjected side (Fig. 5-5). Both injection protocols in that study (6 mL unipedicular, 10 mL bipedicular) resulted in increased strength and restored stiffness to fractured vertebral bodies.

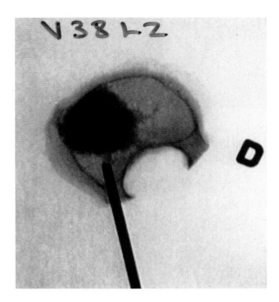

Figure 5-5. Typical distribution of cement after unipedicular injection of 6 mL of PMMA cement.

These results,[36] considered in conjunction with those of the volume-fill study mentioned in the preceding section,[46] suggest that injection of the appropriate cement volume is more important than the manner in which it is injected. Thus, a unipedicular injection of an appropriate volume of cement may allow adequate stabilization with the added benefit of reduced procedure time and risk associated with bilateral cannula placement. A similar ex vivo study[48] compared the compressive strength of vertebral bodies augmented prophylactically by a single posterolateral injection with that of those left unaugmented. Those investigators found that augmentation, even by modest (4.3 ± 1.6 mL) volumes of cement, increased vertebral body strength. Preliminary clinical outcome data on a limited number of patients in which the unipedicular procedure has been performed[45] support the ex vivo findings.[36] It is unknown, however, whether unipedicular injections of volumes used in those ex vivo studies[36,43] would result in adequate mechanical stabilization clinically.

Height Restoration

Restoration of height lost as a result of VCF and correction of the resulting kyphosis have the potential benefit of reducing post-fracture sequelae such as loss of appetite, reduced pulmonary capacity, and diminished quality of life.[49–53] Vertebral body height measured ex vivo suggests that minimal height (i.e., 1–2 mm) is restored after PV.[54–56] To increase height restoration, a new device, the inflatable bone tamp, has been developed.[54,57] The procedure used to place and inflate the bone tamp has been termed *kyphoplasty* (see Chapter 7 for a detailed description). Ex vivo tests indicate that the tamp treatment restores significantly more height than does standard PV treatment and achieves restoration of mechanical properties similar to that of PV.[54,57] A recent report suggests that similar height restoration may be achieved clinically.[58]

Materials and Tests

Cement Alterations

There is no commercially available cement specifically designed for PV. Although Simplex P (Stryker-Howmedica-Osteonics, Rutherford, NJ) has been approved by the Food and Drug Administration (FDA) for use in the treatment of pathological fractures, including those of the spine, its composition (like that of other PMMA cements) is routinely altered to make it better suited to the practice of PV. Common alterations include increasing the monomer-to-polymer ratio to increase working time and decrease viscosity,[13,44,59] adding radiopacifiers to increase cement visualization under fluoroscopy,[13,44,59] and adding antibiotics.[13] Such alterations negate the cement's FDA approval.

Monomer-to-Polymer Ratio

Increasing the monomer-to-polymer ratio decreases the compressive material properties of the cement (Fig. 5-6).[60,61] Because ce-

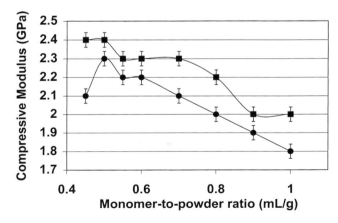

Figure 5-6. Cement compressive modulus as a function of the monomer-to-powder ratio for Simplex P.

ments altered for use with PV typically have monomer-to-polymer ratios of about 0.72 mL/g (compared with the manufacturer-recommended ratio of 0.5 mL/g), there is likely an increased amount of unreacted monomer available to enter the circulatory system.[60,61] Even so, actual blood serum concentration during PV may be lower than that measured during total hip arthrodesis because the quantity of cement injected (< 10 mL) is much smaller than that for hip arthrodesis (> 40 mL).[31,32,62]

Radiopacification

Altering the concentration of radiopacifiers significantly alters the material properties of the cement, as does the combined alteration of monomer-to-polymer ratio and opacification.[63] Although these modifications are statistically significant, they are of dubious clinical importance. In a study of tested cement recipes, the cement composition (Fig. 5-7) that exhibited the minimum relative material properties[63] was the composition that has been used clinically during the past decade in the United States,[13] but there have been no reports of complications associated with mechanical failure of that cement composition. Complications that have been reported are predominantly cement extravasation or the consequences of extravasation.[13,64–66] The prevention of extravasation by means of adequate opacification and careful fluoroscopic visualization during cement injection is essential for the safe practice of PV (Fig. 5-8). Thus, a cement that can be

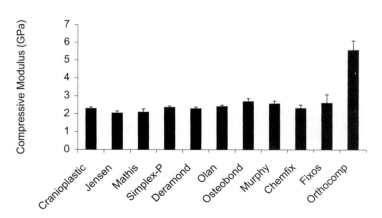

Figure 5-7. Relative compressive strengths for various cement recipes used in PV.

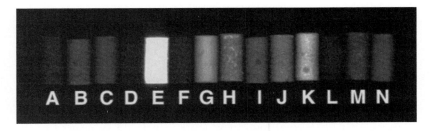

Figure 5-8. Radiopacity of various mixtures of cement: A, Simplex P; B, Simplex P with 20 wt % $BaSO_4$; C, Mathis recipe; D, Cranioplastic with 10 wt % $BaSO_4$; E, Fixos; F, Chemfix3; G, Orthocomp; H, Murphy recipe; I, Olan recipe; J, Simplex P with 30 wt % $BaSO_4$; K, Deramond recipe; L, Cranioplastic with 20% $BaSO_4$; M, Jensen recipe; N, Cranioplastic with 30 wt % $BaSO_4$. (See Jasper et al,[61] for composition details.)

injected easily and has proper opacification takes precedence over a cement that is unmodified and retains its original material properties.

Antibiotics
The efficacy of adding antibiotics to cement to reduce the risk of infection during PV is unknown. In contrast to arthrodesis procedures,[67] the risk of infection from PV is extremely low (< 1 percent). Therefore, elucidating the efficacy of prophylactic antibiotics would require a clinical trial with an extremely large population size for such a study to have sufficient statistical power. For immunocompromised patients, some clinicians routinely add antibiotics to the cement mixture.[13]

It is also unknown what effect adding antibiotics to PMMA cement prepared for PV has on the cement's material properties. The addition of antibiotics to PMMA cement used in arthroplasty reportedly does not affect the cement's fatigue properties[68] and may increase its compressive strength.[67]

Mechanical Tests

Cement Tests
Most mechanical tests for determining the material properties of acrylic bone cements are performed based on Standard F451[69] of the American Society for Testing and Materials (ASTM) or similar test standards. To measure compressive material properties of acrylic cement, the cement components are typically weighed, mixed, and then poured into a mold consisting of cylindrical holes, each 6 mm in diameter and 12 mm high. The mold is placed

between two stainless steel plates and compressed and subsequently placed in a saline (0.09%) bath maintained at 37°C for a given period of time. The cement specimens are sanded flush with the mold, pressed out of the mold, and inspected for defects. Specimens containing defects greater than 10% of their cross-sectional area are culled from the group of test specimens. The specimens are then individually placed between loading platens on a materials testing machine and compressed to failure. Stress and strain data, obtained by dividing the load and deformation data by a specimen's cross-sectional area and initial length, respectively, are plotted for each specimen (Fig. 5-9). Ultimate compressive stress is defined as peak (maximum) stress. Compressive modulus is defined as the slope of the linear (Hookean) portion of the stress–strain curve. Compressive yield strength is determined by means of the 2% offset method, in which a line is drawn parallel to the Hookean portion of the stress–strain curve but offset along the strain axis a distance equal to 2% of the specimen's initial height.

Compression is the loading mode most often used to test cements for PV. Although the cement undoubtedly experiences shear and tensile stresses in vivo, the dominant stress is likely compressive. It is unknown whether cement fatigue is of clinical

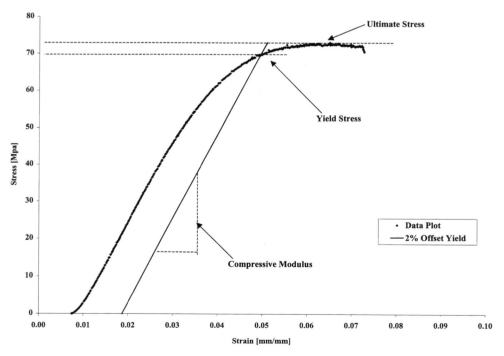

Figure 5-9. Typical compressive material behavior of cement specimens.

concern for the practice of PV. There are no clinical reports describing mechanical failure (fatigue or otherwise) of the cement. Furthermore, it is unknown whether the stress magnitudes, in vivo, are sufficient to cause fatigue. It is unlikely that the stress magnitudes typically experienced by bone cement used with hip arthroplasty are similar to those experienced in the spine. It is also unlikely that the cement used for PV would be exposed to enough cycles to cause fatigue. Most PV is performed on patients advanced in age (> 70 years) whose remaining life span may not be long enough or active enough to elicit a fatigue response. Because of the relatively recent introduction of the practice of PV, there are no patients available for follow-up examinations at more than 15 years after treatment.

Vertebral Body Tests

As with tests conducted on isolated cement specimens, mechanical tests conducted on vertebral bodies to determine their prefracture (initial) and postrepair structural parameters have been almost exclusively compressive.[35,36,46,54] Typically, impressions of the vertebral body end plates are made with a common epoxy to distribute contact stresses across the end plates during compression tests. The potted specimens are placed between loading platens on a materials testing machine and compressed (Fig. 5-10). In this manner, the initial stiffness and failure loads of the vertebral body are determined. Then the particular method under investigation is used to repair the vertebral bodies, and they are recompressed. Strength and stiffness values of the repaired specimens are compared with the initial values to determine the biomechanical effect of the repair (Fig. 5-11).

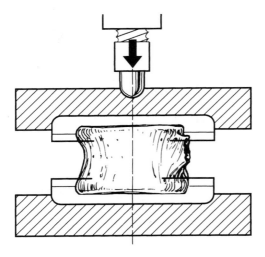

Figure 5-10. Compression test of an osteoporotic vertebral body.

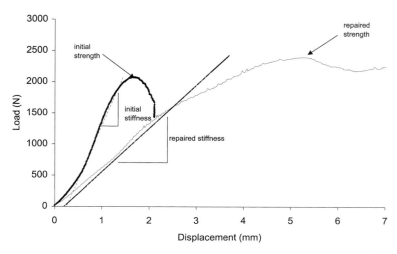

Figure 5-11. Mechanical behavior of an osteoporotic vertebral body during initial compression test and after repair.

Although the spine is loaded predominantly in compression, the effects of bending and torsional loading should not be ignored. Wilson et al.[57] used a multisegment cadaver model to investigate potential altered kinematics as a result of kyphoplasty or PV. Although such models have the benefit of evaluating spine kinematics in a more clinically relevant manner than is possible when one is using isolated specimens, it is difficult in the multisegment model to create the simulated fractures needed to evaluate subsequent repairs. Thus, treatments in the study by Wilson et al.[57] were performed on intact (nonfractured) vertebral bodies, and it is unknown what effect the treatments might have on vertebral bodies mechanically weakened by VCFs.

Alternative Cements

Two factors have motivated the development of new types of cement and injection device: the increasing frequency of the practice of PV and deficiencies in existing PMMA cements for use with PV.[35,70–72] These cements are bioactive or bioresorbable,[70,72,73] are naturally radiopaque,[61,72] and have lower exothermic reactions[28,70,72] than PMMA cements.

Until recently,[56,72] the use of calcium phosphate cements in PV has been substantially impeded by the difficulty of injection of these materials.[70] These more biocompatible cements, however, may eliminate concerns about thermal necrosis and cytotoxicity and appear to result in mechanical stabilization of fractured vertebral bodies similar to that of PMMA.[56,72] Yet, if thermal or chemical mechanisms are found to play an antitumoral role, then the non-PMMA cements may not be as effective for use in patients with tumors. Bioresorbable cements may be most appealing for use in prophylactic augmentation because injected vertebral bodies would be mechanically augmented immediately, whereas the cement would provide an osteoconductive material for subsequent bone repair and remodeling. The subsequent risk of fracture after the cement is remodeled or resorbed is unknown. Bioresorbable cements may also have application with PV for treating burst fractures in young healthy patients.[71] Many questions regarding the clinical use of these cements remain and need to be resolved through careful investigation.

Summary/Conclusions

The practice of PV has experienced explosive growth in recent years, and with it have come many questions regarding the efficacy of the procedure and its optimal practice. Percutaneous vertebroplasty functions primarily to stabilize fractures, thus preventing pain and providing a stable environment for healing. The amount of cement needed to effect stabilization is unknown, but it is probably 4 to 6 mL rather than the volume needed to fill the vertebral body completely (> 10 mL), as previously thought necessary. Altering the cement composition by adding antibiotics, opacifying agents, and more monomers alters the material properties of the cement. The mechanical impact of these alterations is likely to have limited clinical significance, and concern over the alterations should not take precedence over the wish to use a cement that can be properly visualized and easily injected.

References

1. Alleyne CH Jr, Rodts GE Jr, Haid RW. Corpectomy and stabilization with methyl methacrylate in patients with metastatic disease of the spine: a technical note. *J Spinal Disord* 1995; 8(6):439–443.
2. Cortet B, Cotten A, Deprez X, et al. [Value of vertebroplasty combined with surgical decompression in the treatment of aggressive spinal angioma. Apropos of 3 cases.] *Rev Rhum Ed Fr* 1994; 61(1): 16–22.
3. Cybulski GR. Methods of surgical stabilization for metastatic disease of the spine. *Neurosurgery* 1989; 25(2):240–252.
4. Harrington KD. Anterior decompression and stabilization of the spine as a treatment for vertebral collapse and spinal cord compression from metastatic malignancy. *Clin Orthop* 1988; 233:177–197.
5. Harrington KD, Sim FH, Enis JE, et al. Methyl methacrylate as an adjunct in internal fixation of pathological fractures. Experience with three hundred and seventy-five cases. *J Bone Joint Surg* 1976; 58A(8):1047–1155.

6. Mavian GZ, Okulski CJ. Double fixation of metastatic lesions of the lumbar and cervical vertebral bodies utilizing methyl methacrylate compound: report of a case and review of a series of cases. *J Am Osteopath Assoc* 1986; 86(3):153–157.

7. O'Donnell RJ, Springfield DS, Motwani HK, et al. Recurrence of giant-cell tumors of the long bones after curettage and packing with cement. *J Bone Joint Surg* 1994; 76A(12):1827–1833.

8. Persson BM, Ekelund L, Lovdahl R, et al. Favourable results of acrylic cementation for giant cell tumors. *Acta Orthop Scand* 1984; 55(2):209–214.

9. Sundaresan N, Galicich JH, Lane JM, et al. Treatment of neoplastic epidural cord compression by vertebral body resection and stabilization. *J Neurosurg* 1985; 63(5):676–684.

10. Knight G. Paraspinal acrylic inlays in the treatment of cervical and lumbar spondylosis and other conditions. *Lancet* 1959; (ii):147–149.

11. Galibert P, Deramond H, Rosat P, et al. [Preliminary note on the treatment of vertebral angioma by percutaneous acrylic vertebroplasty.] *Neurochirurgie* 1987; 33(2):166–168.

12. Lapras C, Mottolese C, Deruty R, et al. [Percutaneous injection of methyl-methacrylate in osteoporosis and severe vertebral osteolysis (Galibert's technic).] *Ann Chir* 1989; 43(5):371–376.

13. Jensen ME, Evans AJ, Mathis JM, et al. Percutaneous polymethyl methacrylate vertebroplasty in the treatment of osteoporotic vertebral body compression fractures: technical aspects. *Am J Neuroradiol* 1997; 18(10):1897–1904.

14. Cyteval C, Sarrabere MP, Roux JO, et al. Acute osteoporotic vertebral collapse: open study on percutaneous injection of acrylic surgical cement in 20 patients. *Am J Roentgenol* 1999; 173(6):1685–1690.

15. Weill A, Chiras J, Simon JM, et al. Spinal metastases: indications for and results of percutaneous injection of acrylic surgical cement. *Radiology* 1996; 199(1):241–247.

16. Cotten A, Duquesnoy B. Vertebroplasty: current data and future potential. *Rev Rhum Engl Ed* 1997; 64(11):645–649.

17. Bostrom MP, Lane JM. Future directions. Augmentation of osteoporotic vertebral bodies. *Spine* 1997; 22(24 suppl):38S–42S.

18. Deramond H, Depriester C, Galibert P, et al. Percutaneous vertebroplasty with polymethyl methacrylate. Technique, indications, and results. *Radiol Clin North Am* 1998; 36(3):533–546.

19. Lewis G. Properties of acrylic bone cement: state-of-the-art review. *J Biomed Mater Res* 1997; 38(2):155–182.

20. Hasenwinkel JM, Lautenschlager EP, Wixson RL, et al. A novel high-viscosity, two-solution acrylic bone cement: effect of chemical composition on properties. *J Biomed Mater Res* 1999; 47(1):36–45.

21. Leeson MC, Lippitt SB. Thermal aspects of the use of polymethyl methacrylate in large metaphyseal defects in bone. A clinical review and laboratory study. *Clin Orthop* 1993; 295:239–245.

22. Mjoberg B, Pettersson H, Rosenqvist R, et al. Bone cement, thermal injury and the radiolucent zone. *Acta Orthop Scand* 1984; 55(6):597–600.

23. Eriksson RA, Albrektsson T, Magnusson B. Assessment of bone viability after heat trauma. A histological, histochemical and vital mi-

croscopic study in the rabbit. *Scand J Plast Reconstr Surg* 1984; 18(3): 261–268.

24. Rouiller C, Majno G. Morphologische und chemische Untersuchung an Knochen nach Hitzeeinwirkung. *Beitr Pathol Anat Allg Pathol* 1953; 113:100–120.

25. Li S, Chien S, Branemark PI. Heat shock–induced necrosis and apoptosis in osteoblasts. *J Orthop Res* 1999; 17(6):891–899.

26. Jefferiss CD, Lee AJC, Ling RSM. Thermal aspects of self-curing polymethyl methacrylate. *J Bone Joint Surg* 1975; 57B(4):511–518.

27. De Vrind HH, Wondergem J, Haveman J. Hyperthermia-induced damage to rat sciatic nerve assessed in vivo with functional methods and with electrophysiology. *J Neurosci Methods* 1992; 45(3):165–174.

28. Deramond H, Wright NT, Belkoff SM. Temperature elevation caused by bone cement polymerization during vertebroplasty. *Bone* 1999; 25(2 suppl):17S–21S.

29. Cotten A, Dewatre F, Cortet B, et al. Percutaneous vertebroplasty for osteolytic metastases and myeloma: effects of the percentage of lesion filling and the leakage of methyl methacrylate at clinical follow-up. *Radiology* 1996; 200(2):525–530.

30. Dahl OE, Garvik LJ, Lyberg T. Toxic effects of methyl methacrylate monomer on leukocytes and endothelial cells in vitro [published erratum appears in *Acta Orthop Scand* 1995 Aug; 66(4):387]. *Acta Orthop Scand* 1994; 65(2):147–153.

31. Svartling N, Pfaffli P, Tarkkanen L. Blood levels and half-life of methyl methacrylate after tourniquet release during knee arthroplasty. *Arch Orthop Trauma Surg* 1986; 105(1):36–39.

32. Wenda K, Scheuermann H, Weitzel E, et al. Pharmacokinetics of methyl methacrylate monomer during total hip replacement in man. *Arch Orthop Trauma Surg* 1988; 107(5):316–321.

33. San Millan RD, Burkhardt K, Jean B, et al. Pathology findings with acrylic implants. *Bone* 1999; 25(2 suppl):85S–90S.

34. Belkoff SM, Mathis JM, Jasper LE, et al. An ex vivo biomechanical evaluation of a hydroxyapatite cement for use with vertebroplasty. Presented at the Eleventh Interdisciplinary Research Conference on Biomaterials (Groupe de Recherches Interdisciplinaire sur les Biomateriaux Ostéo-articulaires Injectables, GRIBOI), March 8, 2001.

35. Belkoff SM, Mathis JM, Erbe EM, et al. Biomechanical evaluation of a new bone cement for use in vertebroplasty. *Spine* 2000; 25(9):1061–1064.

36. Tohmeh AG, Mathis JM, Fenton DC, et al. Biomechanical efficacy of unipedicular versus bipedicular vertebroplasty for the management of osteoporotic compression fractures. *Spine* 1999; 24(17):1772–1776.

37. Garfin SR, Blair B, Eismont FJ, et al. Thoracic and upper lumbar spine injuries. In: Browner BD, Jupiter JB, Levine AM, et al., eds. *Skeletal Trauma: Fractures, Dislocations, Ligamentous Injuries*. 2nd ed. Philadelphia: WB Saunders Co; 1998:947–1034.

38. Mow VC, Hayes WC. *Basic Orthopaedic Biomechanics*. New York: Raven Press, 1991.

39. WHO Study Group. Assessment of fracture risk and its application to screening for postmenopausal osteoporosis. Report of a WHO Study Group. *World Health Organ Tech Rep Ser* 1994; 843:1–129.

40. Ross PD, Davis JW, Epstein RS, et al. Pre-existing fractures and bone mass predict vertebral fracture incidence in women. *Ann Intern Med* 1991; 114(11):919–923.
41. Eastell R, Cedel SL, Wahner HW, et al. Classification of vertebral fractures. *J Bone Miner Res* 1991; 6(3):207–215.
42. Riggs BL, Melton LJ, III. The worldwide problem of osteoporosis: insights afforded by epidemiology. *Bone* 1995; 17(5 suppl):505S–511S.
43. Lyritis GP, Mayasis B, Tsakalakos N, et al. The natural history of the osteoporotic vertebral fracture. *Clin Rheumatol* 1989; 8(suppl 2): 66–69.
44. Cotten A, Boutry N, Cortet B, et al. Percutaneous vertebroplasty: state of the art. *Radiographics* 1998; 18(2):311–323.
45. Barr JD, Barr MS, Lemley TJ, et al. Percutaneous vertebroplasty for pain relief and spinal stabilization. *Spine* 2000; 25(8):923–928.
46. Belkoff SM, Mathis JM, Jasper LE, et al. The biomechanics of vertebroplasty: the effect of cement volume on mechanical behavior. *Spine* 2001; 26(14):1537–1541.
47. Terjesen T, Apalset K. The influence of different degrees of stiffness of fixation plates on experimental bone healing. *J Orthop Res* 1988; 6(2):293–299.
48. Dean JR, Ison KT, Gishen P. The strengthening effect of percutaneous vertebroplasty. *Clin Radiol* 2000; 55(6):471–476.
49. Lyles KW, Gold DT, Shipp KM, et al. Association of osteoporotic vertebral compression fractures with impaired functional status. *Am J Med* 1993; 94(6):595–601.
50. Silverman SL. The clinical consequences of vertebral compression fracture. *Bone* 1992; 13(suppl 2):S27–S31.
51. Schlaich C, Minne HW, Bruckner T, et al. Reduced pulmonary function in patients with spinal osteoporotic fractures. *Osteoporos Int* 1998; 8(3):261–267.
52. Leech JA, Dulberg C, Kellie S, et al. Relationship of lung function to severity of osteoporosis in women. *Am Rev Respir Dis* 1990; 141(1):68–71.
53. Leidig-Bruckner G, Minne HW, Schlaich C, et al. Clinical grading of spinal osteoporosis: quality of life components and spinal deformity in women with chronic low back pain and women with vertebral osteoporosis. *J Bone Miner Res* 1997; 12(4):663–675.
54. Belkoff SM, Mathis JM, Fenton DC, et al. An ex vivo biomechanical evaluation of an inflatable bone tamp used in the treatment of compression fracture. *Spine* 2001; 26(2):151–156.
55. Belkoff SB, Mathis JM, Deramond H, et al. An ex vivo biomechanical evaluation of a hydroxyapatite cement for use with kyphoplasty. *Am J Neuroradiol* 2001; 22:2212–2216.
56. Belkoff SM, Mathis JM, Jasper LE, et al. An ex vivo biomechanical evaluation of a hydroxyapatite cement for use with vertebroplasty. *Spine* 2001; 26(14):1542–1546.
57. Wilson DR, Myers ER, Mathis JM, et al. Effect of augmentation on the mechanics of vertebral wedge fractures. *Spine* 2000; 25(2):158–165.

58. Lieberman IH, Dudeney S, Reinhardt M-K, et al. Initial outcome and efficacy of kyphoplasty in the treatment of painful osteoporotic vertebral compression fractures. *Spine* 2001; 26(14):1631–1638.

59. Deramond H, Depriester C, Toussaint P, et al. Percutaneous vertebroplasty. *Semin Musculoskelet Radiol* 1997; 1(2):285–295.

60. Jasper LE, Deramond H, Mathis JM, et al. The effect of monomer-to-powder ratio on the material properties of cranioplastic. *Bone* 1999; 25(2 suppl):27S–29S.

61. Jasper LE, Deramond H, Mathis JM, et al. Material properties of various cements for use with vertebroplasty. *J Mate Sci Mate Med* 2002; 13:1–5.

62. Svartling N, Pfaffli P, Tarkkanen L. Methylmethacrylate blood levels in patients with femoral neck fracture. *Arch Orthop Trauma Surg* 1985; 104(4):242–246.

63. Jasper L, Deramond H, Mathis JM, et al. Evaluation of PMMA cements altered for use in vertebroplasty. Presented at the Tenth Interdisciplinary Research Conference on Injectible Biomaterials, Amiens, France, March 14–15, 2000.

64. Padovani B, Kasriel O, Brunner P, et al. Pulmonary embolism caused by acrylic cement: a rare complication of percutaneous vertebroplasty. *Am J Neuroradiol* 1999; 20(3):375–357.

65. Wilkes RA, MacKinnon JG, Thomas WG. Neurological deterioration after cement injection into a vertebral body. *J Bone Joint Surg* 1994; 76B(1):155.

66. Perrin C, Jullien V, Padovani B, et al. [Percutaneous vertebroplasty complicated by pulmonary embolus of acrylic cement.] *Rev Mal Respir* 1999; 16(2):215–217.

67. Saha S, Pal S. Mechanical properties of bone cement: a review. *J Biomed Mater Res* 1984; 18(4):435–462.

68. Riser WH. Introduction. *Vet Pathol* 1975; 12:235–238.

69. American Society for Testing and Materials. Standard F451, Specification for acrylic bone cement. In: *Annual Book of ASTM Standards.* West Conshohocken, PA: American Society for Testing and Materials; 1997:47–53.

70. Schildhauer TA, Bennett AP, Wright TM, et al. Intravertebral body reconstruction with an injectable in situ–setting carbonated apatite: biomechanical evaluation of a minimally invasive technique. *J Orthop Res* 1999; 17(1):67–72.

71. Mermelstein LE, McLain RF, Yerby SA. Reinforcement of thoracolumbar burst fractures with calcium phosphate cement. A biomechanical study. *Spine* 1998; 23(6):664–670.

72. Bai B, Jazrawi LM, Kummer FJ, et al. The use of an injectable, biodegradable calcium phosphate bone substitute for the prophylactic augmentation of osteoporotic vertebrae and the management of vertebral compression fractures. *Spine* 1999; 24(15):1521–1526.

73. Fujita H, Nakamura T, Tamura J, et al. Bioactive bone cement: effect of the amount of glass–ceramic powder on bone-bonding strength. *J Biomed Mater Res* 1998; 40(1):145–152.

6

Procedural Techniques and Materials: Tumors and Osteoporotic Fractures

John M. Mathis

Percutaneous vertebroplasty (PV) is a relatively new procedure that has unique requirements for image guidance, patient preparation, and material selection and utilization. The fast acceptance of PV has driven many changes in the materials now available and in the planned developments to come. This chapter is devoted to the specific requirements that are necessary to the safe and successful performance of PV in osteoporotic vertebral compression fractures (VCFs). Many of these issues are the same for PV performed for the treatment of neoplastic disease. Appendix I (Standard for the Performance of Percutaneous Vertebroplasty by the American College of Radiology) provides additional specifications.

Equipment and Environment

Patient Processing

For the patient's welfare, and to facilitate his or her progress through the preparation, operation, and follow-up procedures, dedicated areas need to be designated for preoperative preparation and postprocedure monitoring. These areas need to be staffed by qualified nursing personnel who are informed about PV and instructed in the scope and presentation of potential side effects.

Procedure Room

Most PV procedures are performed in the hospital setting, in interventional radiology or operating rooms, which are capable of providing sterile environments in which to work. Although a sterile environment is likely beneficial, there are no reports of infection resulting from PV, so such measures are more of a theoretical benefit than an absolute necessity. As in any operative area, room traffic should be minimized, and all personnel should wear clean scrub clothes, caps, and masks. Once the patient has been positioned on the operative table, the anatomical area to be treated should be completely prepared with a full sterile scrub, and the patient should be completely covered with sterile drapes (Fig. 6-1). Equipment in the procedure room (e.g., fluoroscopy tubes) that will come near or in direct contact with the patient or operative team members should also be covered with sterile drapes. A large sterile working environment should be established for needles, syringes, and other materials that will be used during the procedure (Fig. 6-2).

Adequate space needs to be available in the room near the patient's head for nursing or anesthesia personnel to work and care for the patient without being in the way of the operating physi-

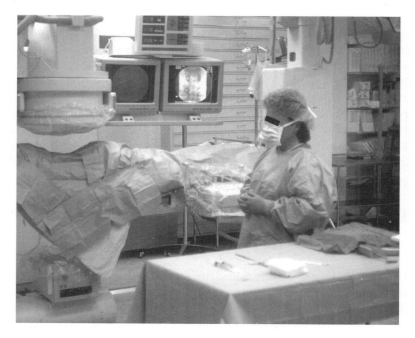

Figure 6-1. Single-plane radiographic room with the patient prone and sterile drapes applied. Full sterile attire is worn.

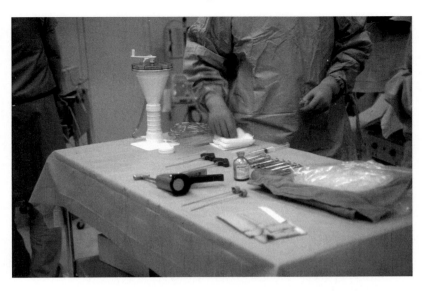

Figure 6-2. A sterile work table, with room for all materials needed for the PV.

cian. In rare circumstances, general anesthesia may be needed. Both space and the necessary connections for the anesthetic machinery must be provided.

At a minimum, monitoring equipment should include devices necessary for continuous heart rate, blood pressure, electrocardiogram (ECG), and oxygen saturation readings. Oxygen should be available and administered as needed. In addition, because the procedure involves conscious sedation (or in rare cases, general anesthesia) and materials that may produce allergic reactions (radiographic contrast or bone cement), pharmaceuticals, devices, and trained personnel capable of managing potential complications with appropriate interventions, including resuscitation, should be available.

In the procedure room, radiographic equipment is essential and should be operated by registered radiology technologists. These individuals should be familiar with all operating aspects of the imaging equipment that is used to perform the PV. It is important that radiographic equipment be adequately comfortable, allowing patients to cooperate fully during the procedure. Poor table padding will result in early patient fatigue and produce unacceptable patient motion. Therefore, the amount of padding found on most angiographic tables should be increased, and extremity supports should be used as needed. Specially developed arm supports (Fig. 6-3) for the prone patient are routinely used.

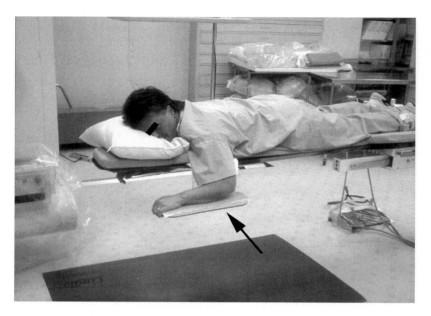

Figure 6-3. Fluoroscopic table with custom-made arm boards (arrow) and additional padding for comfortable prone positioning. These modifications are useful for numerous procedures such as biopsies, discography, and epidural steroid injections.

Image Guidance

Since the first PV procedure,[1] fluoroscopy has been the preferred method of image guidance for performing PV, although computed tomography (CT) has on rare occasions been used as a primary or adjunctive tool.[2,3] Because this procedure was initiated and popularized by interventional neuroradiologists, biplane fluoroscopic equipment was commonly available and often used. This equipment allows multiplanar, real-time visualization for cannula introduction and cement injection and permits rapid alternation between imaging planes without complex equipment moves or projection realignment (Fig. 6-4). However, this type of radiographic equipment is expensive and is not commonly available in interventional suites or operative rooms unless they are used for neurointerventional procedures. Nevertheless, because biplane fluoroscopic equipment facilitates the rapid acquisition of guidance information in two planes, I recommend that the novice operating physician conducting PV use biplane systems initially. If a biplane system is not available, one may be simulated by adding a portable C-arm to the room with a fixed single-plane system, thus creating a temporary biplane configuration that will speed the procedure. In this situation, the equipment that provides the higher quality image should be used for the lateral

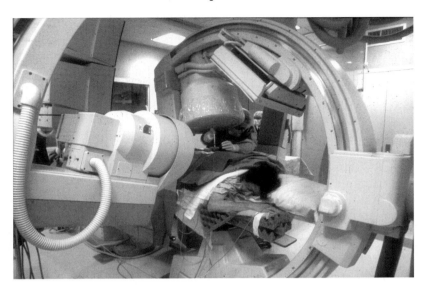

Figure 6-4. Biplanar radiographic room allows visualization in two planes without equipment rotation. This saves time, an advantage that can be essential during cement injection.

projection because that projection is the most critical for monitoring cement injection. This simulated biplane setup may need to be used only until the team becomes familiar with PV and its working efficiency is optimized. The need for speed in the performance of the PV is dictated by the finite working time of the cement once it has been mixed (usually 8–12 min, depending on the cement type and proportions used in the mixture). It takes longer to acquire two-plane guidance and monitoring information with a single-plane than with a biplane system, but it is feasible and safe to use a single-plane fluoroscopic system as long as the operating physician recognizes this necessity for a safe procedure. I commonly use a single-plane system for PV, but I am careful not to accelerate the procedure by watching only in one plane during the needle placement or cement injection.

Gangi et al.[3] introduced the concept of using a combination of CT and fluoroscopy for PV. This method gained a brief period of popularity in the United States with the published study of Barr et al.,[4] but it was later abandoned for routine PV. Although contrast resolution with computerized tomography is superior to that with fluoroscopy, with CT one gives up the ability to monitor needle placement and cement injection in real time. Doing so may be acceptable for needle placement, particularly if a small-gauge guide needle is first placed to ensure accurate and safe location before introducing a large-bore bone biopsy system, but it is certainly not optimum for monitoring the injection of cement.

For this reason, Gangi et al.[3] and Barr et al.[4] used fluoroscopy in the CT suite during cement introduction. Computed tomography does not afford one the opportunity to watch the cement as it is being injected or to alter the injection volume in real time if a leak occurs. Also, unless a large section is scanned with each observation, leaks occurring outside the scan plane may be missed by a physician looking only locally in the middle of the injected body. Barr et al.[4] used general anesthesia with their CT-guided cases because of the need to minimize patient motion. This was successful but added a small additional risk to the procedure and considerable complexity and cost. For all these reasons, CT has not found a primary role in image guidance for PV; it is reserved for extremely difficult cases (see Chapter 9).

Interventions

Laboratory Evaluations

Coagulation tests should be normal, and the patient should not be taking coumadin. Coumadin may be discontinued and replaced with enoxaparin sodium (Lovenox; Rhìne-Poulenc Rorer Pharmaceuticals, Inc., Collegeville, PA), given once or twice a day on an outpatient basis. Coumadin may also be stopped and replaced with heparin, but this medication must be administered intravenously, requiring hospital admission. Both enoxaparin sodium and heparin can be reversed with protamine sulfate before PV and restarted postprocedure. Aspirin use is not a contraindication to the procedure. Percutaneous vertebroplasty is not recommended for patients with signs of active infection, but elevated white blood cell counts clearly associated with medical conditions such as myeloma or secondary to steroid use are not contraindications.

Antibiotics

For PV, as for other surgical procedures that implant devices into the body, intravenous antibiotics are routinely given (usually 30 min) before starting the procedure. The most common antibiotic used in this application is cephazolin (1 g).[5] If an alternative must be used because of allergy, cipro (500 mg orally, two times daily) may be substituted and continued for 24 h after the completion of the procedure. Optimally, an oral antibiotic should be started 12 h before a PV procedure.

An antibiotic (as a powder) may be added to the cement and has been shown to be released over a prolonged interval.[6] The antibiotic most commonly used is tobramycin (1.2 g), and some clinicians routinely add it to the cement.[7] There are no reports of infection in PV, and I have experienced no infections subsequent to PV. For this reason, and because tobramycin powder is very expensive, I do not routinely add antibiotics to the cement. However, because adding antibiotics to bone cement during hip arthroplasty has been shown to reduce infection rates,[8] I do add tobramycin to the cement for use in immunocompromised patients because of their higher risk of infection. An antibiotic may also be considered when there is a question of infection, although one should avoid PV in patients with confirmed infection.

Anesthesia

Whether PV is performed in an inpatient or outpatient setting, it is common to use both local anesthetics and conscious sedation to make the patient comfortable and relaxed. Uncommonly, patients may request not to receive intravenous sedation, and PV may still be accomplished with only mild discomfort if appropriate attention is given to local anesthetic placement. To reduce the sting and discomfort associated with locally administered anesthetics (lidocaine, etc.), one may buffer the material with the addition of a mixture of 1 mL of bicarbonate to 9 mL of lidocaine. This mixture reduces, but does not eliminate, the anesthetic sting. I commonly use a mixture that includes both bicarbonate and Ringer's lactate (Table 6-1), which almost eliminates the sting of the local anesthetic used for procedures such as biopsy and angiography. At my institution, this mixture is prepared daily in the laboratory, and the excess is discarded at the end of each day. This preparation has a low concentration of lidocaine (0.5%) and allows the use of a more generous volume locally with less risk of toxicity.

   Whatever the chosen local anesthetic preparation, the skin, subcutaneous tissues along the expected needle tract, and periosteum of the bone at the bone entry site must be thoroughly infiltrated. If this is accomplished before the needle introduction, the patient will experience only mild discomfort while the bone needle is being placed, regardless of whether conscious sedation is used.

TABLE 6-1 Modified Local Anesthetic Solutions

Solution	Local anesthetic type (mL)[a]			
	Lidocaine (4%)	Lactated Ringer's	Bicarbonate	Epinephrine
1[b]	4	24	2	0
2[c]	4	24	2	0.15 (1:1000)

[a]These solutions should be mixed daily and discarded at the end of the day. The total volume of each mix is 30 mL.

[b]Makes a "sting-free" local anesthetic with 0.5% lidocaine.

[c]Is "sting-free" with 0.5% lidocaine and 1:200,000 epinephrine.

Conscious sedation has become a common adjunctive method of pain and anxiety control in awake patients who undergo minimally invasive procedures. I use a combination of intravenous midazolam (Versed, Roche; Manati, PR) and fentanyl (Sublimase, Abbott Labs; Chicago). It may be helpful to begin these medications before the patient is placed on the operative table to decrease anxiety and diminish the discomfort associated with positioning. Dosages are chosen according to patient size and medical condition. The final amount is determined with titration while observing the patient's response.

General anesthesia is rarely needed for PV, but it is used occasionally for patients in extreme pain who cannot tolerate the prone position used in PV or for patients with psychological restrictions that preclude a conscious procedure. It is not needed for routine PV and should be avoided when possible because it adds a mild risk and considerable cost to the procedure. As described earlier, Barr et al.[4] used general anesthesia routinely with CT-guided procedures to ensure minimum patient motion.

Needle Introduction and Placement

The original choice of a device for percutaneous cement introduction was based on device availability.[1,9] The French group used a 10-gauge beveled needle with no handle (introduced with a small mallet); the American group used an 11-gauge Jamshidi bone biopsy trocar and cannula with an affixed handle that obviated the need of a hammer. The size of these devices was empirically chosen to allow the injection of viscous polymethylmethacrylate (PMMA) cement. It was quickly discovered that a small (1- or 3-mL) syringe is necessary to gain the hydraulic advantage needed to push the cement into the intertrabecular space of the vertebral marrow while displacing marrow and fat elements. In addition, the cement mix was altered to make it more liquid. However, a disadvantage of "liquefying" the cement was that it could more easily leak out of the vertebra and thereby cause potential complications (indicating that cement should always be used at maximal viscosity). This was particularly true if the needle tip was placed in the posterior half of the vertebral body. In this area, there is a confluence of large veins that communicate directly with the epidural venous plexus and provide a direct route for cement leak (Fig. 6-5). This anatomical feature of the vertebra led my colleagues and me routinely to position the needle tip in the ventral half of the body before injecting cement. Access was typically made via transpedicular approach, a technique that was popularized by Galibert et al.[1]

The original PV procedure has been modified as new tech-

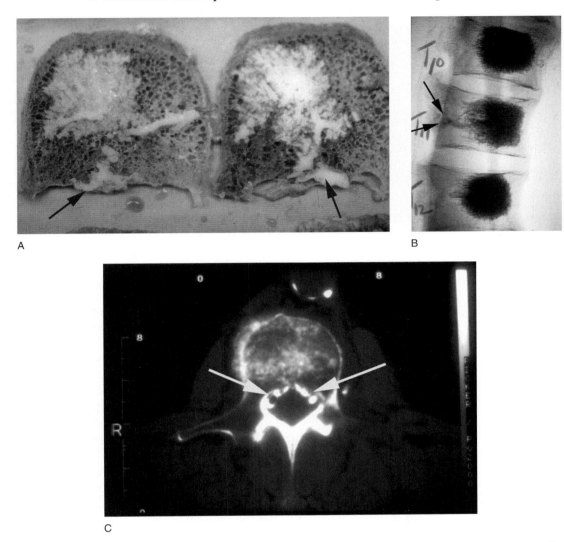

A

B

C

Figure 6-5. Cement leakage. (A) Microtome section of osteoporotic cadaver vertebra partially filled with PMMA, showing a leak of cement (arrows) through the posterior confluens of veins into the epidural space, which occurred even though the epicenter of the injection was anterior to the midline of the vertebra. (B) Lateral view of T11 showing a leak of cement (arrows) through the posterior confluens, even though the injection was well anterior to the midline. (C) A CT scan postinjection showing cement leaking (arrows) into the epidural space through the posterior venous confluens.

niques and materials have been developed. For example, several new trocar and cannula systems have been developed for the percutaneous delivery of cement (Fig. 6-6A). Although these devices are approved by the Food and Drug Administration (FDA) for bone biopsy, no device has yet been approved specifically for PV.

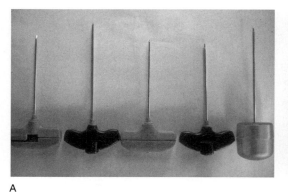
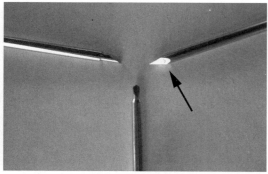

A   B

Figure 6-6. Trocar–cannula systems successfully used for percutaneous cement delivery. (A) The handles of these systems are not detachable. (B) Of the various tip geometries available, the sharp point (arrow) with the trocar ground to match the cannula seems to work best.

These systems have in common a large-bore (10- to 11-gauge) central removable trocar, fixed handle, and various tip geometries. The handle variations offer little real difference between needle types; all provide adequate purchase for hand introduction. Many operating physicians now choose to use a mallet for introduction because it may offer more control, but I still introduce the needle with slow, rotary hand pressure. In my experience, it seems to produce less patient discomfort. The tip geometries (Fig. 6-6B) all work well, and therefore the choice is more a matter of personal preference than of actual difference in function. Several of the cannulae are tapered (larger at the hub than at the tip), but such tapering has two disadvantages: (1) the trocar fits tightly only at the tip, leaving considerable dead space in the proximal part of the needle, and (2) a trocar cannot be used as a plunger to discharge the residual cement from the cannula, a technique that is very useful when the cement becomes viscous and difficult to inject.

Several introductory routes for needle delivery are possible, including transpedicular, parapedicular (transcostovertebral), posterolateral (lumbar only), and anterolateral (cervical only). The classical route for most PV is transpedicular. It offers the following advantages: (1) it usually provides the operating physician with a definite anatomic landmark for needle targeting (Fig. 6-7); (2) it is very effective for PV and for biopsy of lesions inside the vertebral body; and (3) it is inherently safe, with no other adjacent anatomic structures that might be damaged with the needle (i.e., nerve root, lung, etc.) as long as an intrapedicular location is maintained.

In the upper thoracic region and in small patients, the size of the pedicle may be too narrow for an 11-gauge needle. In this

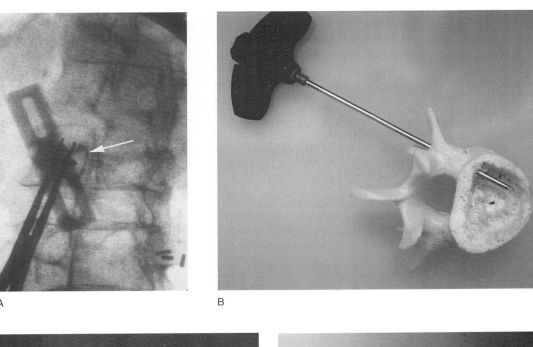

A   B

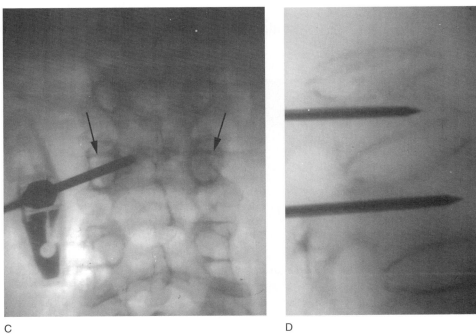
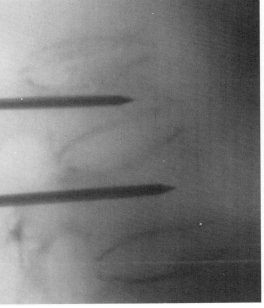

C   D

Figure 6-7. The transpedicular route. (A) An oblique fluoroscopic image showing the insertion of a trocar–cannula system (arrow, cortical wall of pedicle). (B) Sawbone model showing typical transpedicular needle approach. The tip of the needle is usually constrained more toward the lateral edge of the vertebral body with this method. (C) AP view showing the needle in the vertebral body (arrows, pedicle cortices). (D) Lateral view showing needles in place in two vertebra. The tip of each needle is anterior to the midline of the associated vertebra, a good starting position for cement injection.

situation, a 13-gauge needle may be used. This smaller needle increases the difficulty of cement injection, but the result is an acceptable trade-off. One potential disadvantage of the transpedicular route is that there is relatively little latitude for placing the needle tip in the vertebral body and yet keeping the needle within the pedicle. The pedicle has an almost AP direction in the thoracic and upper lumbar spine. Therefore, except in wide pedicles and at L5, following the pedicle will constrain the needle to a lateral position within the vertebral body. This position is quite safe for injection but may not offer good filling across the midline of the vertebral body with a single injection.

The parapedicular or transcostovertebral approach (Fig. 6-8) was devised to address several of the shortcomings of the transpedicular route described earlier. First, because the needle passes along the lateral aspect of the pedicle, rather than through it, a small pedicle is not restrictive for an 11-gauge needle for cement introduction. Also, this approach angles the needle tip more toward the center of the vertebral body than does the transpedicular approach. At least in theory, this angle may allow easier filling of the vertebra with a single injection. The disadvantage is that a central needle position, if at or behind the midline in the vertebra, increases the likelihood that cement will flow quickly

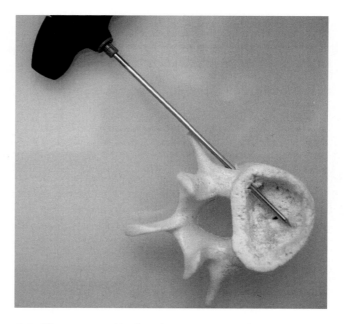

Figure 6-8. The parapedicular (transcostovertebral) approach. This sawbone model shows the needle entry adjacent to (not below) the pedicle. With this trajectory, it is easier to place the needle tip near the vertebral midline for a single injection.

into the large posterior venous plexus and into the epidural space. One may reduce this risk by keeping the needle tip in the anterior third of the body when injecting. Finally, a parapedicular approach needs to hug the lateral aspect of the pedicle because a more lateral position, in the thoracic spine, increases the risk of puncturing the lung and creating a pneumothorax. A potential problem with the parapedicular route (and the posterolateral approach described below) is that the needle enters the body only through the lateral wall. This procedure may increase the risk of cement leakage through the hole when the needle is removed. However, I believe this risk is low as long as the needle is retracted after the cement begins to harden. This is almost always the case with the faster polymerizing cements but not with the slow-set types (e.g., Cranioplastic, Depuy International, Ltd., trading as CMW; Blackpool, England).

The posterolateral approach has a trajectory similar to that of the parapedicular approach, but the needle usually enters the vertebra more inferiorly and only through the lateral wall. It is an approach historically used for Craig needle biopsies.[10] Because the needle traverses a route that can easily intersect the nerve root that exits under the pedicle, it can potentially produce immediate pain and persistent nerve damage. I believe this route is of historical interest only, and I do not use it.

In the cervical spine, a transpedicular route is very difficult, so an anterolateral approach may be used as an alternative. Needle introduction must avoid the carotid–jugular complex. To accomplish this goal, the operating physician (as in cervical discography) manually pushes the carotid out of path of the needle. Alternatively, CT can be used to visualize the carotid, and a trajectory that will miss the vascular structures can then be chosen. A small guide needle can be inserted to ensure accurate placement outside the carotid complex. I prefer the guide needle alternative because it gives positive guidance and confirmation without excessive fluoroscopy to my hands during needle introduction. However, because osteoporotic fractures in this area are rare, the cervical spine only occasionally undergoes PV. Neoplastic disease may produce an occasional need for PV intervention in the cervical spine.

Once the needle route has been chosen, local anesthesia is administered, and a small dermatotomy incision is made with a number 11 scalpel blade. The trocar-and-cannula system is introduced through the skin and subcutaneous tissue to the periosteum of the bone. This introduction can be facilitated with a sterile clamp to guide the needle during fluoroscopy, thus avoiding radiation to the operating physician's hands (Fig. 6-9). In osteoporotic bone, penetrating the bone cortex and advancing the needle into the body is usually very easy. In a patient with neo-

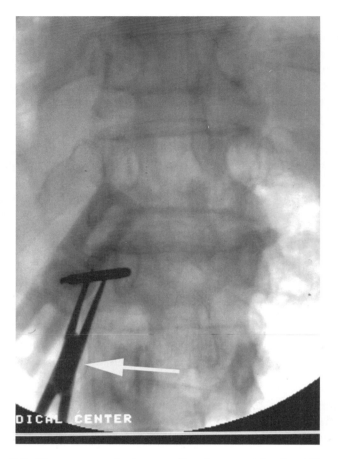

Figure 6-9. Fluoroscopy during needle placement in the AP and AP oblique projections can be accomplished without fluoroscopy to the operating physician's hands by using a clamp (arrow) as a needle-holding device.

plastic disease, the bone may be very dense and strong (except where it has been destroyed by a tumor), and in this situation, the use of a mallet to advance the needle is a technique clearly superior to that of manual advancement. Regardless of whether a transpedicular or parapedicular route has been chosen, the tip of the needle should lie anterior to the vertebral midline as viewed from the lateral projection. I usually try to obtain an even more anterior position by starting at the junction of the anterior and middle thirds (Fig 6-7D).

Venography

The need for, and utility of, venography in PV procedures have become somewhat controversial issues. In Europe, venography is not often associated with PV, but in the United States, venography has been used by some clinicians in an attempt to predict potential cement leaks. In my experience and opinion, using venography with PV presents several disadvantages. First, the concept of injecting radiographic contrast medium through the cannula before injecting the cement is logical, but its predictive value is flawed by the extreme difference in the flow characteristics of radiographic contrast medium and bone cement. Unlike viscous cement, contrast flows like water and follows the vascular pattern through the marrow with rapid efflux into the paraspinous and epidural venous plexus, to the vena cava, and into the lungs (Fig. 6-10A). This pathway happens in all cases of injected contrast, even when subsequent cement injection proves to be safe, with good filling of intertrabecular space (Fig. 6-10B). Second, those who use venography rarely make substantial changes in their injection methods based on the findings of venography. Third, venography increases the cost of PV, requires

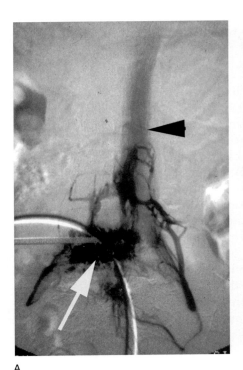
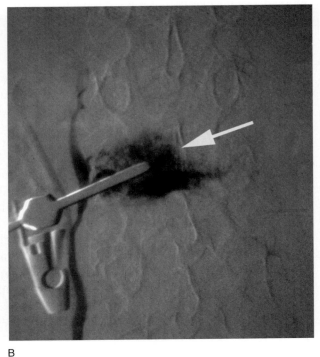

A   B

Figure 6-10. Venography of osteoporotic vertebral body. (A) Normal L5 contrast venogram showing filling of a normal-appearing trabecular space (white arrow), epidural and paraspinous veins, and the inferior vena cava (black arrowhead). This is not an abnormal or dangerous venogram. It simply shows the filling that can occur with the injection of too much cement. (B) Early-phase contrast venogram showing a normal intraosseous (intertrabecular) stain (arrow) and secondary filling of a paraspinous vein.

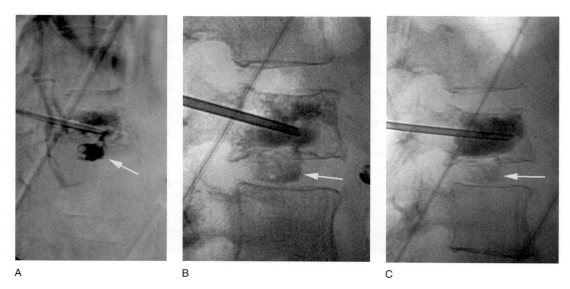

A   B   C

Figure 6-11. Vertebral venography. (A) A lateral subtraction image showing a contrast leak into the subjacent disk space (arrow). (B) Cement injection. Because the contrast could not be washed out with a saline injection (arrow), it hindered visualization through out the PV and made it difficult to ensure that cement did not leak into the disk as well. (C) Final image showing good vertebral filling with no leak of cement into the disk space (arrow).

the patient to be injected with contrast material, and exposes all involved to radiation. Fourth, I believe the use of venography adds no real beneficial information and is, at times, a detriment. For example, in the presence of a fracture of the vertebral end plate, contrast will commonly extravasate into the disk during venography (Fig. 6-11A).[7] Because a disk is basically avascular, the contrast medium cannot be easily flushed with saline, and the resulting obscurity makes it difficult or impossible to determine possible cement leakage into this space during injection (Fig. 6-11B). The fact that contrast leaks into the disk does not mean that cement will (Fig. 6-11C). Unlike contrast in disks, contrast that fills a vertebral cavity can be partially washed out with a saline infusion, lessening the contrast's masking effect.

To summarize, venography may be considered to be a basically safe procedure, but I believe it offers no intrinsic safety to performing PV, and at times it can hinder visualization of cement injection. Therefore, I stopped using venography with PV in 1995; doing so has not resulted in decreased safety or increased complications.

Cement Selection, Opacification, and Introduction

Currently, the only cements used for PV are PMMA-based compounds of various types. The first cement used for PV was

Simplex P (Stryker-Howmedica-Osteonics, Rutherford, NJ). This was and still is the most popular cement for PV in Europe. In the United States, a PMMA cement approved as a cranial void filler (Cranioplastic) has been commonly used. These two cements are used for most PV procedures. Although no PMMA has named approval for PV by the FDA, Simplex P is approved for treating pathological fractures anywhere in the body. No other PMMA has approval for use in the spine. Cranioplastic is not intended as a structural cement but rather as a cranial defect filler. My colleagues and I originally used Cranioplastic,[5,9,11] but I have switched completely to Simplex P and do not modify the ratio of powder (copolymer) to liquid (monomer) during cement preparation (see exact mixing procedure shortly). Crucial to performing PV safely is the accurate monitoring of cement injection in real time.[11] Such monitoring is usually accomplished with fluoroscopy, which requires that the cement be opacified so that small quantities may be visualized.

Cements intended for orthopedic reconstruction often have barium sulfate added as an opacifier for radiographic evaluation. This is true of Simplex P, which contains 10% barium sulfate by weight. This percentage allows standard radiographic examination of the large quantities used in arthroplasty, but it is insufficient for fluoroscopic visualization of the small quantities used in PV (Fig. 6-12A). Indeed, the safety of the procedure seems closely linked to being able to visualize the cement well during injection. In clinical practice and in laboratory evaluations, it has been determined that fluoroscopic visualization requires approximately 30% barium sulfate by weight (Fig. 6-12B). However, changing the amount of barium sulfate in PMMA can have definite effects on the structural characteristics of PMMA (see details in Chapter 5).[12,13]

Biomechanical evaluations of these cements in cadaver spines indicate that PV generally increases strength and restores stiffness of vertebral bodies. Although there are substantial differences in material properties between the various cements, cement material properties play only a partial role in structural repair of VCF with PV. The volume of cement injected and the density of the host bone are also factors that determine repair strength (see Chapter 5).

Most physicians performing PV have indicated that they modify the liquid-to-powder (monomer-to-polymer) ratio of the cement to decrease viscosity and prolong the liquid (or injectable) phase or "working time." There are some potential disadvantages of altering the monomer-to-polymer ratio. First, PMMA cements are treated as devices by the FDA, and any alteration in the monomer-to-copolymer ratio changes the device,[14] and thus its approval. Some authors have incorrectly suggested that this

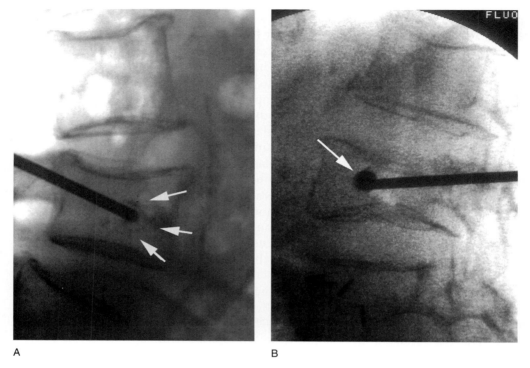

Figure 6-12. Cement opacification. (A) 10% barium sulfate cannot be well visualized under fluoroscopy (arrows). (B) Fluoroscopy can accurately monitor cement opacified with 30% barium sulfate (arrow).

modification is simply an "off-label use"[7]; off-label use would be to use the unmodified cement in a location or application for which it is not approved. Second, altering this monomer-to-polymer ratio not only changes the cement's mechanical properties, it may also increase the unbound monomer (liquid) content available to circulate throughout the body. Third, this material is toxic and in large quantities may produce hypotension as well as cardiac and/or neurological dysfunction. All the above-mentioned issues (regulatory problems, changes in cement structure, and toxicity) have led me to use and recommend a cement preparation that attempts to alter the cement as little as possible from the manufacturer's specifications.

As mentioned, I now use Simplex P. I add 10 g of sterile barium sulfate to the original powder and monomer proportions provided in the cement package, bringing the total barium sulfate quantity to 25 wt %. No other alteration is made. The monomer is chilled (4°C) for 24 h before the procedure and is removed from the cold environment only when ready for mixing. Mixing is performed in a vacuum chamber provided by the cement manufacturer. Care must be taken during transfers of cement to maintain sterility. The cement holding chamber is kept cold by wrapping it in a sterile cold pack, which prolongs the cement's polymerization time. This method allows a working time of 8 to 10 min to be achieved with no modification of the monomer-to-copolymer ratio.

Cement injection is accomplished via 1-mL syringes; a complex and expensive injection device is not necessary. The syringes can be filled in a closed fashion directly from the chilled cement holding chamber. These syringes should not be filled until ready for injection because warming the cement to room temperature hastens polymerization. The cement should be tested to ensure that it is thickening (it should never be used when it is liquid enough to drip from the syringe tip). Injection should be gradual to allow visualization and control; rapid injection often creates patient discomfort and patient motion. Real-time fluoroscopic monitoring should be used during injection, or one should inject a small quantity of cement (0.1–0.2 mL) and image to see the result before injecting more. Both methods allow the operating physician ample time to see extravasation of cement and to terminate the injection, if necessary. Incremental injection of small volumes seems to be better tolerated by the awake patient because it allows intraosseous pressure to normalize, relieving any pain that may be created by injection. Visualization is primarily in the lateral projection to ensure early detection of any cement that may leak into the epidural space, inferior vena cava, or disk space. Intermittent visualization in the AP direction is needed to see any lateral leak.

As the cement continues to thicken, it may become difficult to inject. An alternative method is to insert the trocar into the cannula and use it as a plunger, which is more effective for very viscous cement than an injection device. This procedure should be performed slowly with monitoring because a 4-in., 11-gauge cannula can contain up to 0.7 mL of cement that will be delivered once the trocar has been fully introduced into the cannula. Longer cannulae may contain greater amounts of cement. If more cement is needed, the trocar can be removed and the cannula can again be loaded with the 1-mL syringe. The procedure can be repeated as needed to obtain adequate filling.

The amount of vertebral filling needed to obtain pain relief is not known. Originally, operating physicians tried to achieve as complete a fill as possible without leakage (Fig. 6-13). However, no clinical studies are available that correlate amount of cement or degree of filling with pain relief. Indeed, Cotten et al.[15] have suggested that no correlation exists. An ex vivo study has suggested that volumes between 4 and 8 mL may be sufficient for

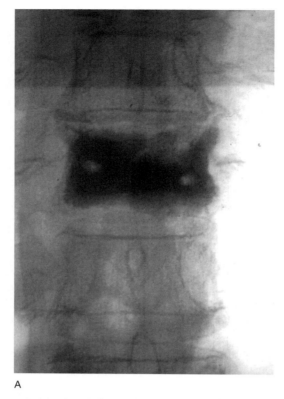

A

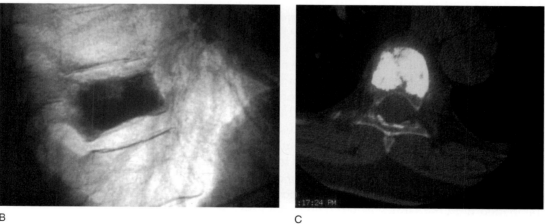

B   C

Figure 6-13. Example of early excessive filling: (A) lateral view, (B) AP view, and (C) CT scan.

restoring vertebral mechanical properties, depending on the vertebral level injected.[16] These volumes are considerably smaller than those used in many early cases (often 8–12 mL).[9] Today, filling volumes are typically smaller, but they provide similar pain control with a lower risk of cement leak (Fig. 6-14).[4] One should

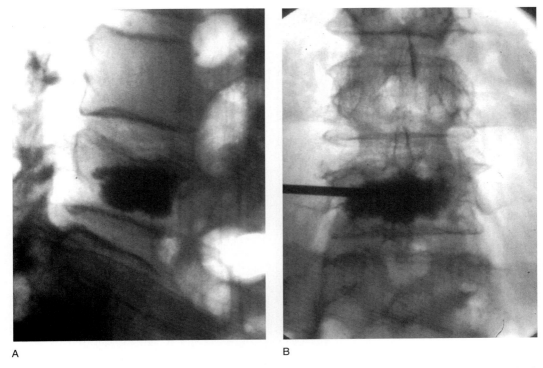

Figure 6-14. This vertebral cement fill was adequate, resulting in good pain relief and no leaks. (A) Lateral view. (B) AP view.

be aware that not all vertebrae fill uniformly when injected (Figs. 6-15 and 6-16). This lack of uniformity makes a less-than-desirable radiographic example of PV, but its result is usually as good as that from a uniform fill.

I still routinely place two needles in each vertebra and then mix the cement. I use both needles to fill a vertebra, finishing with one needle before beginning the second. This guarantees good filling of a vertebra with a single cement mix, regardless of the spread of cement from any single needle. Some operating physicians use only one needle to perform PV.[4] Single-needle injections work well in many cases, provided the cement crosses the midline of the vertebra. However, if a single injection of cement is not adequate, a second needle must be placed and a second batch of cement mixed. This increases procedure time, and patients do not tolerate the procedure as well as when both needles are placed at the same time. Ex vivo data suggest that it is not necessary to fill both sides of the vertebra to obtain effective reinforcement (Fig. 6-17).[17]

Once the cement has been injected, the cannula can be removed. With bilateral cannulae, one should not be removed be-

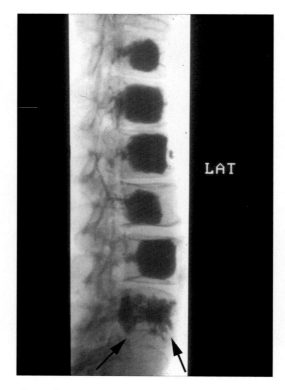

Figure 6-15. Lateral view of a cadaver spine with multiple vertebra filled with the same cement. All fills are homogeneous except the lowest, indicated by a very irregular fill pattern (arrows).

fore the other is filled. Premature removal may allow leakage of the cement into the pedicle or cannula entry site while the second cannula is being injected. Rotating the cannula several times in place will disconnect the cement at the cannula tip from that in the vertebra. The cannula may then be removed without the risk of depositing a column of cement in the soft tissues.

When the cannula is extracted, it is not uncommon to get fairly brisk venous bleeding from the puncture site. This bleeding is easily controlled with local pressure for 3 to 5 min. Failure to apply pressure can result in a local hematoma, bruising, and excessive local postprocedure tenderness. The puncture site should be cleaned, and Betadine ointment should be applied locally. The site should then be covered with a sterile bandage or occlusive dressing. This dressing may be removed in 24 h; the area should be kept clean and dry for 48 h. After that time, no special treatment is needed if there is no excessive redness, swelling, or drainage.

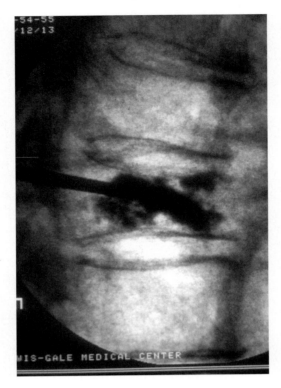

Figure 6-16. Lateral view showing an irregular fill pattern. Nevertheless, the patient had a good clinical result.

Postprocedure Care

In Europe, it is still common to keep patients overnight after PV. This practice was the standard initially in the United States as well. In 1995, at the University of Maryland, I started performing PV as an outpatient procedure on all ambulatory patients because inpatient care seemed to be limited to observation and bed rest. Performing this procedure on an outpatient basis reduced its cost, has been well accepted by patients, and has not been associated with delayed complications.

At the completion of the PV, the patient is maintained recumbent and moved from the radiographic or operative table to a stretcher. For the first hour, the patient should remain supine. Polymethylmethacrylate cements typically attain 90% of their maximal strength within 1 h.[18] During this interval, the patient's vital signs are checked at 15-min intervals. The patient is also assessed for neurological change or dysfunction, especially in the lower extremities, because most PVs are performed in the mid-thoracic spine or lower. A pain assessment is performed because

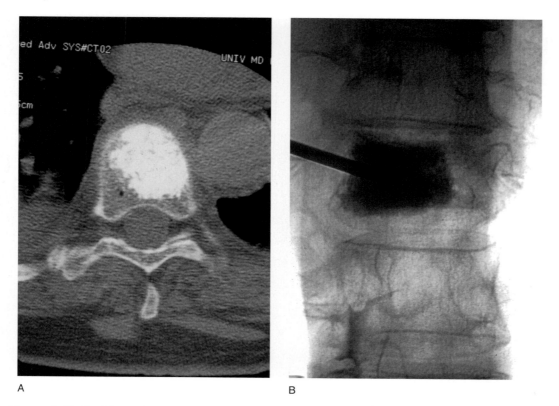

A   B

Figure 6-17. In this patient, unipedicular injection provided filling across the midline and substantially filled the vertebra. (A) CT scan. (B) AP view.

a few patients may experience an increase in local pain after PV. The pain is usually self-limiting, but it may require therapy with parenteral or narcotic analgesics as well as nonsteroidal antiinflammatory medications. If the pain is severe, the patient may need short-term hospitalization for management. Neurological changes or increased pain should initiate an immediate search for a source of the pain, including a CT scan of the treated area to visualize possible cement extravasation. A concurrent surgical consult should also be obtained. This pain syndrome may be idiopathic, but that is a diagnosis of exclusion. All surgical problems need to be immediately eliminated.

If no complications are noted in the first hour, the patient is allowed to sit up and may begin ambulation after 2 h. Nursing assessments are continued. After 2 h of uneventful observation, the patient may be discharged to the care of another adult who will be available to provide care for the next 24 h (see Table 6-2 for sample postprocedure care and discharge procedures). Relief of pain after PV usually occurs within 4 to 48 h postprocedure.

TABLE 6-2 **Sample Postprocedure Orders and Discharge Instructions**

Postprocedure

Bed rest 1 h postprocedure (may roll side to side).

May sit up after 1 h with assistance.

Vital signs and neurological examinations (focused on the lower extremities) every 15 min for the first hour, then every 30 min for the second hour.

Record pain level (visual analog scale, 1–10) at end of procedure and at 2 h postprocedure (before discharge). Compare with baseline values and notify physician if pain increases above baseline.

May have liquids by mouth if no nausea.

Discontinue oxygen (if used) after procedure (if saturation is normal).

Discontinue intravenous drips after 1 h if recovery is otherwise uneventful.

Discharge patient home with adult companion after 2 h if recovery is uneventful.

Discharge

Return home; bed rest or minimal activity for next 24 h.

May resume regular diet and medications.

Keep operative site covered for 24 h. Bandages may then be removed and site washed with a damp cloth. Do not soak.

Notify physician/facility in the event of increasing pain, redness, swelling, or drainage from the operative site.

Notify physician/facility in the event of new difficulty walking, changes in sensation in the hips or legs, new pain, or problems with bowel or bladder function.

The area of the procedure will be tender to the touch for 24 to 48 h. This is to be expected.

If pain similar to that before the procedure continues, prescribed pain medications may be continued as needed.

However, the patient may need to continue prescribed analgesics during this time. It is recommended that a telephone follow-up call be made to the patient 1 to 7 days postprocedure to assess the response to PV. This information is helpful for the operating physician and for the institution in maintaining outcome data for quality improvement.

All patients who have experienced an osteoporotic VCF need to be placed in the care of a physician who can assess the level of osteoporosis and administer therapeutic medications in an attempt to counteract additional bone mineral loss. Lifestyle changes may need to be instituted to prevent future osteoporosis-related fractures.

Summary/Conclusions

The practice of PV requires high-quality imaging equipment and a trained staff. The use of biplane fluoroscopy is preferred, but with care the procedure may be performed with single-plane fluoroscopy. Care must be exercised when placing the needles to avoid injuring adjacent nerves or vessels. Cement should be visualized during injection to prevent extravasation and potential complications. Percutaneous vertebroplasty is a safe and minimally invasive procedure that can be performed on an outpatient basis; patients are typically discharged 2 h after the procedure.

References

1. Galibert P, Deramond H, Rosat P, et al. [Preliminary note on the treatment of vertebral angioma by percutaneous acrylic vertebroplasty.] *Neurochirurgie* 1987; 33(2):166–168.
2. Barr JD, Barr MS, Lemley TJ. CT as the sole imaging modality for performance of percutaneous vertebroplasty. Poster presented at the 36th Annual Meeting of the American Society of Neuroradiology, Philadelphia, May 17–21, 1998.
3. Gangi A, Kastler BA, Dietemann JL. Percutaneous vertebroplasty guided by a combination of CT and fluoroscopy. *Am J Neuroradiol* 1994; 15(1):83–86.
4. Barr JD, Barr MS, Lemley TJ, et al. Percutaneous vertebroplasty for pain relief and spinal stabilization. *Spine* 2000; 25(8):923–928.
5. Mathis JM, Petri M, Naff N. Percutaneous vertebroplasty treatment of steroid-induced osteoporotic compression fractures. *Arthritis Rheum* 1998; 41(1):171–175.
6. Eckman JB, Jr, Henry SL, Mangino PD, et al. Wound and serum levels of tobramycin with the prophylactic use of tobramycin-impregnated polymethylmethacrylate beads in compound fractures. *Clin Orthop* 1988; 237:213–215.
7. Jensen ME, Dion JE. Percutaneous vertebroplasty in the treatment of osteoporotic compression fractures. *Neuroimaging Clin North Am* 2000; 10(3):547–568.
8. Norden CW. Antibiotic prophylaxis in orthopedic surgery. *Rev Infect Dis* 1991; (13 suppl)10(4):S842–S846.
9. Jensen ME, Evans AJ, Mathis JM, et al. Percutaneous polymethyl methacrylate vertebroplasty in the treatment of osteoporotic vertebral body compression fractures: technical aspects. *Am J Neuroradiol* 1997; 18(10):1897–1904.
10. Craig FS. Vertebral-body biopsy. *J Bone Joint Surg* 1956; 38A(1):93–102.
11. Mathis JM, Eckel TS, Belkoff SM, et al. Percutaneous vertebroplasty: a therapeutic option for pain associated with vertebral compression fracture. *J Back Musculoskel Rehab* 1999; 13(1):11–17.
12. Belkoff SM, Maroney M, Fenton DC, et al. An in vitro biomechanical evaluation of bone cements used in percutaneous vertebroplasty. *Bone* 1999; 25(2 suppl):23S–26S.
13. Jasper L, Deramond H, Mathis JM, et al. Evaluation of PMMA cements altered for use in vertebroplasty. Presented at the Tenth Interdisciplinary Research Conference on Injectible Biomaterials, Amiens, France, March 14–15, 2000.

14. Jasper LE, Deramond H, Mathis JM, et al. The effect of monomer-to-powder ratio on the material properties of Cranioplastic. *Bone* 1999; 25(2 suppl):27S–29S.
15. Cotten A, Dewatre F, Cortet B, et al. Percutaneous vertebroplasty for osteolytic metastases and myeloma: effects of the percentage of lesion filling and the leakage of methyl methacrylate at clinical follow-up. *Radiology* 1996; 200(2):525–530.
16. Belkoff SM, Mathis JM, Jasper LE, et al. The biomechanics of vertebroplasty: the effect of cement volume on mechanical behavior. *Spine* 2001; 26(14):1537–1541.
17. Tohmeh AG, Mathis JM, Fenton DC, et al. Biomechanical efficacy of unipedicular versus bipedicular vertebroplasty for the management of osteoporotic compression fractures. *Spine* 1999; 24(17):1772–1776.
18. Jasper LE, Deramond H, Mathis JM, et al. Material properties of various cements for use with vertebroplasty. *J Mate Sci Mate Med* 2002; 13:1–5.

7

Balloon Kyphoplasty

Wade H. Wong, Wayne J. Olan, and Stephen M. Belkoff

Percutaneous vertebroplasty (PV) reportedly achieves relief of pain from vertebral compression fractures (VCFs) in 70 to 90% of cases,[1–4] but it does not address the kyphotic deformity that typically results from VCFs. Kyphosis can cause difficulties on multiple fronts. Biomechanically, kyphosis shifts the patient's center of gravity forward, rendering the patient off-balance and at increased risk for a fall and subsequent and potentially more debilitating injury. A change in a patient's center of gravity also creates additional stress on the vertebrae, increasing the risk of fracture.[5]

Kyphosis caused by compression fractures in the lumbar or thoracic region decreases vital capacity in the lungs, thus accentuating restrictive lung disease.[6] Leech et al.[7] reported a 9% average decrease in forced vital capacity per osteoporotic compression fracture in the thoracic region. In addition, fractures in both the thoracic and lumbar spine can lead to gastrointestinal difficulties. Increasing kyphosis may cause the ribs to increase pressure on the abdomen, creating a sensation of bloating that may lead to early satiety, decreased appetite, and malnutrition.[8] It is therefore not surprising that both retrospective and prospective studies have demonstrated decreased life expectancy in patients who have sustained VCFs. In a retrospective study, Cooper et al.[9] found that the 5-year survival rate for patients with VCFs was lower than that for patients with hip fractures. A prospective study by Kado et al.[10] showed that patients with VCFs had a 23% increase in mortality compared with age-matched controls. The increased mortality was postulated to result from possible

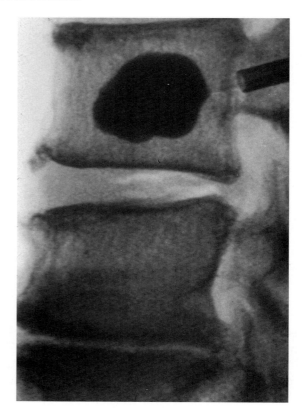

Figure 7-1. Lateral view of inflated bone tamps used to elevate col-lapsed vertebral body end plates.

pulmonary causes, including pneumonia and chronic obstructive pulmonary disease, accentuated by the effects of the kyphosis.

In an attempt not only to reduce or eliminate the pain of VCFs, but also to improve or prevent the resultant kyphotic deformity, a new procedure, termed kyphoplasty, has been developed. This procedure consists of inserting a balloonlike device percutaneously into a compressed vertebral body, inflating the device, and thereby elevating the end plates and restoring vertebral body height (Fig. 7-1). Theoretically, this procedure would be expected both to im-prove vital lung capacity, appetite, and longevity and to reduce the likelihood of additional falls or refractures.

Patient Selection

Selection criteria for patients to undergo kyphoplasty are similar to those for PV. As with PV, the patient selection process includes obtaining the patient's history and a physical examination, preferably with fluoroscopic localization of the fractured level, and a magnetic resonance (MR) image showing fracture deformity with marrow edema. Additional imaging studies may be necessary.

Kyphoplasty is usually used to treat osteoporotic VCFs, although it has also been used in patients with vertebral body involvement from neoplastic disease processes such as plasmocytoma or multiple myeloma. The likelihood of restoring vertebral body height depends largely on the density of the bone. In our experience, less dense or weaker cancellous bone is more likely to be encountered in patients with recent VCFs (usually < 3–6 months old) or in patients with ongoing secondary osteoporosis (e.g., those undergoing steroid therapy).

The exclusion criteria for balloon kyphoplasty are also very similar to those used for PV: (1) VCFs that are not painful or are not the primary source of pain or (2) the presence of osteomyelitis or systemic infection, retropulsed bone fragments, or a posterior tumor mass that may seriously compromise the spinal canal.

Pretreatment detection of retropulsed bone fragments (Fig. 7-2) or posterior tumor mass (Fig. 7-3) must be a priority because these entities could be forced into the spinal canal during balloon inflation. In addition, there must be sufficient residual height for the instruments used with kyphoplasty to be inserted into the compressed vertebral body. Thus, although PV may be performed in a severely compressed vertebral body, kyphoplasty of the same vertebral body may not be technically feasible. In ad-

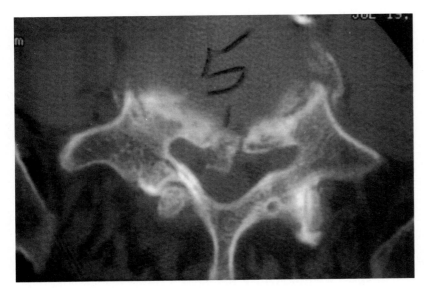

Figure 7-2. An axial CT image showing a retropulsed bony fragment and fracture line. This patient was not considered to be a candidate for kyphoplasty or PV.

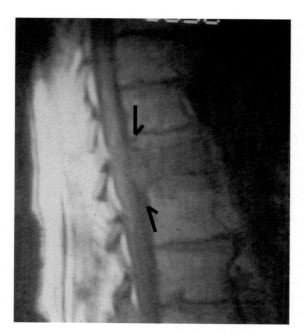

Figure 7-3. A tumor (arrows) extending from the vertebral body and compromising the canal is a contraindication to kyphoplasty.

dition, small pedicles may also be a limiting factor because the instruments used for kyphoplasty are somewhat larger than those for PV. Kyphoplasty can be performed safely from L5 to T7 in most patients, although in some cases it has been performed at higher levels.[11]

Technique

The kyphoplasty technique is very similar to that of PV. The patient is positioned on the fluoroscopic operating table in a prone position, with the arms extended cranially and the hands resting comfortably underneath the forehead. With the arms in this position, it is important to avoid an antecubital intravenous line. The elbows are taped in position to avoid elbow "flop" and potential injury by a rotating fluoroscope.

High-resolution C-arm or biplane fluoroscopy must be used when the kyphoplasty procedure is performed. The patient is positioned so that the spine is located at isocenter of the C-arm. The fracture is then identified fluoroscopically. The approach is usually bilateral transpedicular; however, a single posterolateral approach can be used for the large lower lumbar vertebrae (almost always at L5; less commonly at L2-L4). An extrapedicular approach must be used when the pedicles are too small to accommodate the kyphoplasty instruments (usually in the mid- or upper thoracic regions).

Localization of the pedicles is performed in a manner similar to that used for PV. A posterior approach with slight ipsilateral obliquity of 10° to 25° is preferred. The medial wall of the pedicle must be well visualized. The patient's overlying skin is then marked with indelible ink before sterile cleansing.

After the patient has been sterilely prepared and draped, and after the fluoroscopy equipment has also been sterilely covered, local anesthetic is injected, typically with a 25-gauge needle; however, if a longer needle is needed, a spinal needle can be used. Most patients require only local anesthesia and conscious sedation. As in PV, the key to local anesthesia is extension of the anesthetic to the periosteum of the pedicle. Patients who cannot lie in a prone position may be candidates for general anesthesia. Prophylactic antibiotics are administered.

The kyphoplasty procedure requires an 11- or 13-gauge (4- or 6-in., respectively) bone entry needle, a scalpel, a kyphoplasty kit (Fig. 7-4), inflatable balloon tamps, sterile barium sulfate or other opacifier, and polymethylmethacrylate (PMMA) cement. The procedure is begun by directing the entry needle into the bone under fluoroscopic guidance (Fig. 7-5). For a transpedicular approach, the needle is directed through the pedicle to the poste-

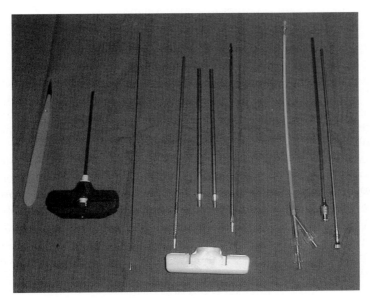

Figure 7-4. The kyphoplasty kit consists of scalpel, 11-gauge needle, K-wire, blunt dissector, two cannulae, drill, handle, inflatable balloon tamp, bone filler device, and angioplasty inflator (not shown here: see Fig. 7-9).

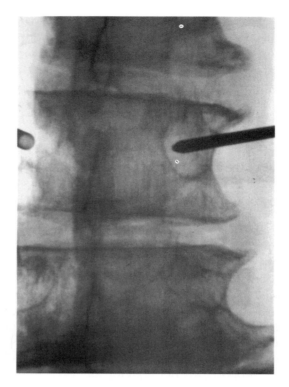

Figure 7-5. With lateral-to-medial angulation, the pedicle is seen on end. In this illustration, a bone entry needle is being placed by the transpedicular approach with lateral to medial angulation.

rior aspect of the vertebral body. For very small pedicles, an extrapedicular approach can be used that involves targeting a starting point just superior and lateral to the pedicle (almost costovertebral in the thoracic region). If a single posterolateral approach is chosen, the trajectory can be established along a posterolateral path similar to that used for discography. This approach is appropriate for the larger lumbar vertebrae, especially L5. One must be cautious to avoid injuring the exiting nerve roots; the beginning point must not be so far lateral that the bowel or kidney is endangered. When the posterolateral approach is used, the drill should cross the midline of the vertebra on AP and lateral views. Oblique views should also be used to confirm proper positioning. The advantage of the single posterolateral approach is the time saved by placing only one balloon instead of two; the disadvantage is a reduction of the working surface area of the inflatable balloon tamp.

The trocar of the needle is removed. A Kirschner wire (K-wire) is then directed through the needle and into the bone, and the needle cannula is removed. A blunt dissector is then fitted over the K-wire and directed under fluoroscopic guidance into the bone to be situated at the level of the K-wire (Fig. 7-6). In the case of a transpedicular approach, the K-wires and blunt dissector are directed to the posterior third of the vertebral body. One should manipulate the K-wire with the same caution one would use for a guidewire in the vascular system. The operating physician should always have control of the proximal end of the K-wire because the sharp tip could easily penetrate soft bone and breach the anterior vertebral cortex.

A skin incision is then made to accommodate the working cannula, which is advanced through the soft tissues over the blunt dissector and through the pedicle to rest along the posterior aspect of the vertebral body. A plastic handle can be placed on the hub of the cannula to advance it manually into the vertebral body if the bone is sufficiently easy to penetrate, or a mallet can be used to tap the plastic handle, driving the cannula into the vertebral body. If there is considerable resistance to placing the working cannula, the cannula's handle can be rotated in an alternatingly clockwise, counterclockwise (screwing) motion to help breach the cortex and facilitate advancement. When using the

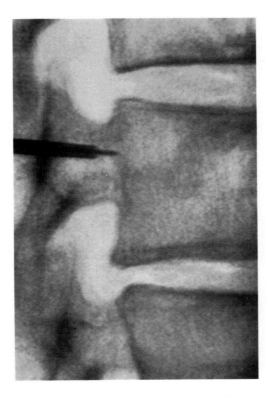

Figure 7-6. The blunt dissector positioned over the K-wire, entering the posterior part of the vertebral body.

mallet, one must be careful to direct the blows onto the handle; inadvertently striking the K-wire or the blunt dissector might drive the piece deeper into the vertebra.

Next, the K-wire and the blunt dissector are removed, leaving the working cannula in place. A 3-mm drill is advanced through the cannula, and multiplanar fluoroscopy is used to recheck the orientation of the working cannula. Then the drill is directed ideally along a slightly posterolateral-to-anteromedial trajectory into the vertebra until the tip of the drill is 3 to 4 mm posterior to the anterior margin of the vertebral body, or at least within the anterior third of the vertebral body (Fig. 7-7). If the fracture involves the superior aspect of the vertebral body, the drill must be directed somewhat inferiorly to the midline of the vertebral body. If the fracture is along the inferior aspect of the vertebra, then the drill must be directed superiorly to the midline of the vertebra. Extreme caution should be used to avoid breaching the anterior cortex of the vertebral body with the drill. For bilateral transpedicular or extrapedicular approaches, the sequence of events is repeated on the contralateral side.

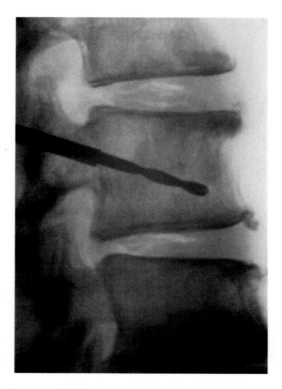

Figure 7-7. A 3-mm drill placed through the working cannula created a cavity extending into the anterior third of the vertebral body.

The inflatable balloon tamp is available in different sizes. Each balloon has markers to delineate its distal and proximal extents (Fig. 7-8). These markers are also radiopaque and easily visualized under fluoroscopy. The tamps are then prepared for inflation. Air is purged from the balloons, and the reservoir of an angioplasty injection device (incorporating a pressure monitor) is filled with 10 mL of diluted iodine contrast (Fig. 7-9). If the patient has an allergy to iodine, gadolinium can be substituted. The drill is then removed. (If there is a question of underlying malignancy, a biopsy can be effectively performed by pushing the drill bit back and forth in the cavity to collect bone fragments, before the drill is removed from the working cannula.)

The uninflated balloon tamps are inserted through the working cannulae under fluoroscopy and directed to the most anterior extent of the vertebral body. If the clinician feels resistance in the passageway of the drilled hole, perhaps secondary to small shards of bone, the drill or bone filler device can be inserted and withdrawn once or twice along the path to clear it of debris, and the balloon tamp can then be inserted without difficulty.

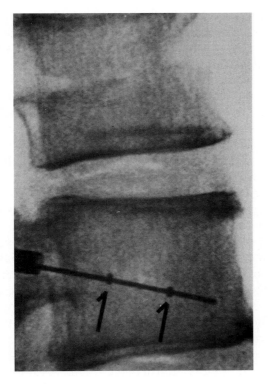

Figure 7-8. An inflatable balloon tamp placed within the cavity created by a drill. Arrows on the two fiducial markers denote the proximal and distal extents of the balloon.

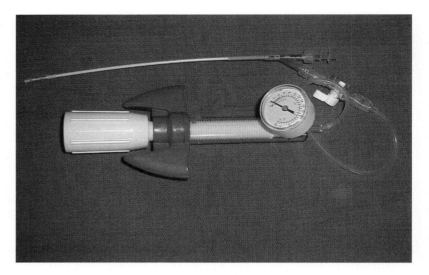

Figure 7-9. Inflatable balloon tamp with angioplasty inflation device.

Balloon inflation should be performed slowly, not rapidly. Inflation via the injection device is begun under continuous fluoroscopy, increasing balloon pressure to approximately 50 psi to secure the balloon in position. The stiffening wire is withdrawn from the shaft of the tamps, and the contrast media volume in the reservoir is recorded. The balloons are progressively inflated by 0.5-mL increments (Fig 7-10), with frequent pauses to check for pressure decay, which occurs as the adjacent cancellous bone yields and compacts. If the bone is osteoporotic, immediate decay may occur. If the bone is quite dense, then little or no decay may occur, even at pressures up to 180 psi. The balloon system is rated to 180 psi, with a practical maximum of 220 psi. Even with slow inflation, pressures higher than 220 psi have been achieved in dense bone. If a balloon ruptures, it is simply withdrawn through the working cannula and replaced.

The end point of inflation can be restoration of the vertebral body height to normal, flattening of the balloon against an end plate without accompanying height restoration, contact with a lateral cortical margin, inflation without further pressure decay, or reaching the maximum volume of the balloon or maximum pressure. The operating physician must maintain both visual and manual control throughout the entire inflation process and should record the amount of fluid used to inflate the balloon when the end point has been achieved. This volume indicates the size of the cavity that has been created, and it will serve as an estimate of the amount of cement to be delivered. If substantial

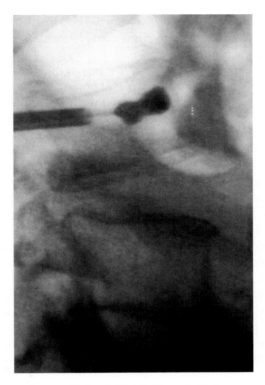

Figure 7-10. Initial balloon inflation.

height restoration has not been achieved, careful repositioning of the tamps and followed by reinflation may be helpful.

Once adequate inflation has been achieved, the cement is mixed in a manner similar to that for PV. The cement mixture is transferred to a 10-mL syringe that is used to fill a series of 1.5-mL bone filler devices. The volume of cement for injection is approximately 1 mL more than the volume of the cavity created by each inflatable balloon tamp. Once the bone cement has transitioned from a liquid to a cohesive, doughy consistency (about 3–4 min after mixing), the bone filler devices are passed through the working cannula and into the anterior aspect of the vertebral cavities. The cavity is then filled with cement in a retrograde fashion while continuous monitoring for leakage of cement into the spinal canal, paraspinous veins, inferior vena cava, or disk space is maintained with lateral fluoroscopic visualization. One potential technical advantage of kyphoplasty compared with PV may be the ease of low-pressure cement delivery into the cavity created by the inflatable balloon tamp, although delivery of the final milliliter (that in excess of cavity size) requires higher pressures, similar to those used in PV. Some operating physicians prefer to fill one cavity first, leaving the contralateral balloon inflated as a supporting strut. This maneuver may be effective at maintaining height elevation.

When cement filling of the cavity has been confirmed fluoroscopically from both lateral (Fig. 7-11) and anteroposterior views, the bone filler devices are withdrawn partially to allow complete filling of the cavity; they are used to tamp the bone cement in place before being withdrawn completely. The cannulae are then rotated (so they are not cemented in the bone) and removed, and hemostasis is obtained at the incision site using manual pressure. Steri-Strips are usually sufficient for wound closure. The patient remains prone on the table and is not moved until the remaining cement in the mixing bowl has hardened completely. The usual time frame for kyphoplasty is 35 to 45 min, which compares favorably with the 25 to 35 min per level required for PV. In harder bone, the balloons may take longer to respond to small incremental increases in pressure.

The follow-up and postoperative procedures for kyphoplasty are identical to those for VB. At some institutions, kyphoplasty and PV are performed on an outpatient basis unless the patient is extremely frail, or unless the procedure is performed at the end of the day and staffing issues make it easier to keep the patient overnight for discharge the next morning. Outpatients are observed for 3 to 4 h after the procedure.

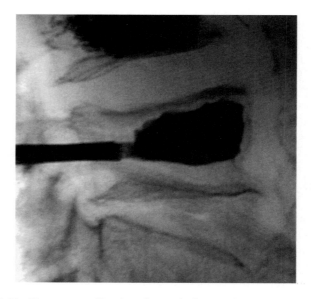

Figure 7-11. Cement application through the working cannula with the bone filler tube. Note the smooth margins of the low-pressure cement application within the cavity created by the balloon. The vertebral body above it showed the more feathered margins typical of PV.

It must be noted that kyphoplasty is a technically demanding surgical procedure. Safe performance requires a high level of skill and high-quality imaging equipment. One should not perform this procedure without being an expert in clinical and radiographic spinal anatomy, without having completed a kyphoplasty course with expert instructors, and without imaging equipment that is capable of clearly delineating key bony landmarks, particularly the pedicles, the cortices, and the spinous processes.

Results

Kyphoplasty is a relatively new procedure and, as such, peer-reviewed literature reporting clinical results are few. One early outcome study of 70 vertebral bodies treated in 30 patients reported average restoration of lost height of 2.9 mm.[11] When the treated vertebrae were separated into two groups, 70% gained an average of 4.1 mm (46.8% height restoration), whereas 30% gained no height. Cement extravasation occurred in 8.6% of the levels treated, a rate similar to that reported for PV used for osteoporotic VCFs (see Chapter 10). The findings of this initial report were consistent with preliminary results reported at various professional meetings. In one report, the average vertebral body height restoration of 24 procedures performed was as follows: anterior, 3.7 mm; middle, 4.7 mm; and posterior, 1.5 mm.[12] There was good to excellent pain relief in every case, and no complications were reported. Lane et al.[13] reported on 30 patients with similar height restorations and pain relief, and a complication rate of less than 1%. The complications included one episode of epidural bleeding requiring surgical decompression, one incomplete spinal cord injury, and one transient case of adult respiratory distress syndrome.

These early clinical reports are encouraging. A long-term follow-up study needs to be conducted to determine the theoretically beneficial effect of height restoration on pulmonary function, quality of life, and the prevention of kyphosis. Furthermore, the pain relief obtained after kyphoplasty is similar to that reported for PV. Although the exact mechanism of pain relief is unknown, it is likely that for both procedures it is the fracture stabilization obtained by the cement injection. A randomized prospective clinical trial comparing kyphoplasty with PV is needed to answer such questions.

Biomechanical Investigations

The magnitude of height restoration mentioned in the preliminary clinical reports discussed earlier is similar to those measured ex vivo.[14] In the ex vivo study by Belkoff et al.,[14] average actual height restoration (average of six height measurements made circumferentially about the vertebral body) was 2.5 ± 0.7 mm. Furthermore, ex vivo tests have suggested that compared with standard PV treatment, the tamp treatment restores significantly more height and achieves similar mechanical restoration.[14,15] Other reports indicate that height restoration has the potential benefit of reducing postfracture kyphosis and its associated sequelae.[6–8,16,17] It is important to note that an ex vivo study of osteoporotic vertebral bodies that were compressed to create simulated fractures and repaired with PV suggested that half of the compressed height recovers elastically,[14] a phenomenon similar to that reported in vivo.[18] In addition, 30% of the height that was not elastically recovered in ex vivo specimens was restored by using PV, whereas kyphoplasty restored 97%.[14] The actual height restoration seems to range from 2.5 to 3.5 mm, values similar to those reported clinically.[11]

One of the theoretical advantages of kyphoplasty compared with standard PV is that the former permits the injection of cement under lower pressures, a factor that is particularly important for the use of calcium phosphate and hydroxyapatite cements, which are bioresorbable but difficult to inject.[19–23] A recent ex vivo study comparing a hydroxyapatite-forming cement and a PMMA cement found that height restorations were similar and that the cements were qualitatively as easy to inject, but the former produced a weaker and less stiff repair than that produced by PMMA.[24] Another ex vivo study in which the same hydroxyapatite cement was directly injected into osteoporotic vertebral bodies substantiated the finding that this class of cements are similarly easy to inject as PMMA cements.[24] Thus, it appears that the ease of injection of the hydroxyapatite cement may have more to do with its composition than with the environment into which it is injected. Injection pressure was not measured in either study.

Summary/Conclusions

Kyphoplasty seems to ameliorate the pain of osteoporotic and malignant VCFs with a success rate similar to that of PV. However, kyphoplasty may also provide an opportunity for restoring vertebral body height before stabilization and reduction of a fracture in the clinical setting. These hypotheses need to be tested by a prospective clinical trial in which patients are randomly assigned to kyphoplasty and PV treatment groups. An ongoing randomized clinical trial is under way to compare kyphoplasty with conventional medical management of VCFs.

References

1. Galibert P, Deramond H, Rosat P, et al. [Preliminary note on the treatment of vertebral angioma by percutaneous acrylic vertebroplasty.] *Neurochirurgie* 1987; 33(2):166–168.
2. Jensen ME, Evans AJ, Mathis JM, et al. Percutaneous polymethylmethacrylate vertebroplasty in the treatment of osteoporotic vertebral body compression fractures: technical aspects. *Am J Neuroradiol* 1997; 18(10):1897–1904.
3. Gangi A, Kastler BA, Dietemann JL. Percutaneous vertebroplasty guided by a combination of CT and fluoroscopy. *Am J Neuroradiol* 1994; 15(1):83–86.
4. Cotten A, Dewatre F, Cortet B, et al. Percutaneous vertebroplasty for osteolytic metastases and myeloma: effects of the percentage of lesion filling and the leakage of methyl methacrylate at clinical follow-up. *Radiology* 1996; 200(2):525–530.
5. White AA, Panjabi MM. *Clinical Biomechanics of the Spine*. 2nd ed. Philadelphia: JB Lippincott Co; 1990.
6. Schlaich C, Minne HW, Bruckner T, et al. Reduced pulmonary function in patients with spinal osteoporotic fractures. *Osteoporos Int* 1998; 8(3):261–271.
7. Leech JA, Dulberg C, Kellie S, et al. Relationship of lung function to severity of osteoporosis in women. *Am Rev Respir Dis* 1990; 141(1): 68–71.
8. Silverman SL. The clinical consequences of vertebral compression fracture. *Bone* 1992; 13(suppl 2):S27–S31.
9. Cooper C, Atkinson EJ, O'Fallon WM, et al. Incidence of clinically diagnosed vertebral fractures: a population-based study in Rochester, Minnesota, 1985–1989. *J Bone Miner Res* 1992; 7(2):221–227.
10. Kado DM, Browner WS, Palermo L, et al. Vertebral fractures and mortality in older women: a prospective study. Study of Osteoporotic Fractures Research Group. *Arch Intern Med* 1999; 159(11): 1215–1220.
11. Lieberman IH, Dudeney S, Reinhardt M-K, et al. Initial outcome and efficacy of kyphoplasty in the treatment of painful osteoporotic vertebral compression fractures. *Spine* 2001; 26(14):1631–1638.
12. Theodorou DJ, Wong WH, Duncan TD, et al. Percutaneous balloon kyphoplasty: a novel technique for reducing pain and spinal deformity associated with osteoporotic vertebral compression fractures [abstract]. *Radiology* 2000; 217(suppl):511.
13. Lane JM, Girardi F, Parvaianen H, et al. Preliminary outcomes of the first 226 consecutive kyphoplasties for the fixation of painful osteoporotic vertebral compression fractures [abstract]. Osteoporosis Int 2000; (suppl):11:S206.
14. Belkoff SM, Mathis JM, Fenton DC, et al. An ex vivo biomechanical evaluation of an inflatable bone tamp used in the treatment of compression fracture. *Spine* 2001; 26(2):151–156.
15. Wilson DR, Myers ER, Mathis JM, et al. Effect of augmentation on the mechanics of vertebral wedge fractures. *Spine* 2000; 25(2):158–165.
16. Lyles KW, Gold DT, Shipp KM, et al. Association of osteoporotic

vertebral compression fractures with impaired functional status. *Am J Med* 1993; 94(6):595–601.

17. Leidig-Bruckner G, Minne HW, Schlaich C, et al. Clinical grading of spinal osteoporosis: quality of life components and spinal deformity in women with chronic low back pain and women with vertebral osteoporosis. *J Bone Miner Res* 1997; 12(4):663–675.

18. Nelson DA, Kleerekoper M, Peterson EL. Reversal of vertebral deformities in osteoporosis: measurement error or "rebound"? *J Bone Miner Res* 1994; 9(7):977–982.

19. Schildhauer TA, Bennett AP, Wright TM, et al. Intravertebral body reconstruction with an injectable in situ–setting carbonated apatite: biomechanical evaluation of a minimally invasive technique. *J Orthop Res* 1999; 17(1):67–72.

20. Belkoff SM, Mathis JM, Erbe EM, et al. Biomechanical evaluation of a new bone cement for use in vertebroplasty. *Spine* 2000; 25(9): 1061–1064.

21. Mermelstein LE, McLain RF, Yerby SA. Reinforcement of thoracolumbar burst fractures with calcium phosphate cement. A biomechanical study. *Spine* 1998; 23(6):664–670.

22. Bai B, Jazrawi LM, Kummer FJ, et al. The use of an injectable, biodegradable calcium phosphate bone substitute for the prophylactic augmentation of osteoporotic vertebrae and the management of vertebral compression fractures. *Spine* 1999; 24(15):1521–1526.

23. Cunin G, Boissonnet H, Petite H, et al. Experimental vertebroplasty using osteoconductive granular material. *Spine* 2000; 25(9):1070–1076.

24. Belkoff SB, Mathis JM, Deramond H, et al. An ex-vivo biomechanical evaluation of a hydroxyapatite cement for use with kyphoplasty. *Am J Neuroradiol* 2001; 22:1212–1216.

8

Tumors

Osteolytic metastases and myeloma are the most frequent malignant destructive lesions involving the spine. Affected patients
often experience severe back pain and disability related to the
vertebral fractures induced by these destructive lesions. The aim
of percutaneous vertebroplasty (PV) in these disease processes is
to produce pain relief and reinforcement by the injection of acrylic
cement. This treatment may be used adjunctively with radiation
therapy and chemotherapy.

Percutaneous vertebroplasty is rarely indicated for benign tumors. Spinal osteoid osteoma can be treated by other percutaneous methods[1] but not by PV. Spinal aneurysmal bone cysts do
not need structural reinforcement and therefore are not an indication for PV, although they can be treated by percutaneous
chemoablation.[2] Fibrous dysplasias, eosinophilic granulomas,
and vertebral hemangiomas (VHs) are lesions that weaken bone,
and PV has been used in their treatment.[3–5] The most frequent
indication for PV in the treatment of benign tumors is VH.

This chapter describes the role of PV in the treatment of malignant tumors, myelomas, and VHs.

Part I: Metastatic Tumors

Hervé Deramond, Claude Depriester,
and Jacques Chiras

Pathology and Patient Demographics

Patients with cancer ultimately present with bone metastases in
27% of cases.[6] The vertebral bodies are the most common site of
bone metastatic disease.[7] The incidence of metastatic lesions to

the spine depends on the primary cancer: 80% of patients with prostate cancer, 50% of patients with breast cancer, and 30% of patients with lung, thyroid, or renal cell cancer.[8] Breast (30%), prostate (10%), and lung (25%) cancers are the three main etiologies of metastases to the spine.[7,8]

The one-year survival after diagnosis of spinal metastases is high for patients with prostate (83%) or breast (78%) cancer (hormonal-dependent cancers) but low in patients with lung cancer (22%).[9] Survival rates in patients with renal cell or thyroid cancer depend on the histological classification of the tumor cells.[9] The detection of spinal metastasis from the time of primary lesion diagnosis is shortest in patients with lung cancer (3.6–6.1 months) and longest in patients with breast cancer (29.4–33.5 months); 7.5% of patients present with spinal metastases before the diagnosis of the primary lesion.[10] These data are important to consider when counseling patients for therapy.

Indications and Contraindications

The primary indication for PV is proven metastatic disease to the spine of a patient who is experiencing severe, focal, and mechanical back pain that limits normal activities and requires narcotic medications. Usually there will be a vertebral compression fracture (VCF) associated with the metastatic lesion, although the amount of compression may be small.

Inherent in the process of malignant involvement of the spine is destruction of portions of the vertebral body. The greater the destruction, the more chance there is for vertebral collapse and pain. In addition, these lesions present problems for the physician considering PV because destruction of the cortex of the vertebra, although not a contraindication, increases the possibility of cement leak. In several series, 40% of patients treated with PV had partial destruction of the posterior wall (Fig. 8-1).[11–13] However, there are considerations that are unique to this situation. If there is extension of the tumor through the posterior wall (Fig. 8-2), PV should be used only after a multidisciplinary discussion, and a surgical team should be available in case spinal cord decompression is needed after PV. Clinical signs of compression of nerve roots or cord are contraindications to PV because there is a distinct risk of increasing compression with the injection of cement.

In general, PV is not indicated for asymptomatic lesions of the spine. One should first consider other therapies (radiotherapy, chemotherapy, thermoablation, etc.). Percutaneous vertebroplasty can be performed if other therapies have been exhausted and/or if there is a high risk of vertebral collapse (Fig. 8-3).

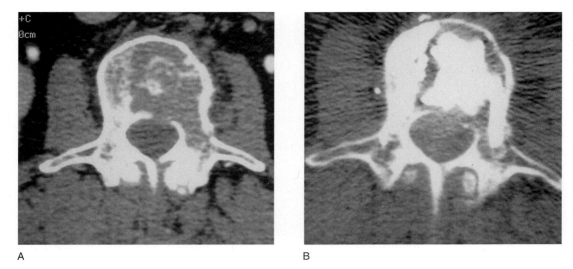

A   B

Figure 8-1. Partial destruction of the posterior wall. Axial CT scans before (A) and after (B) injection of cement. Note the injection of both the "normal" part and osteolytic part of the vertebral body.

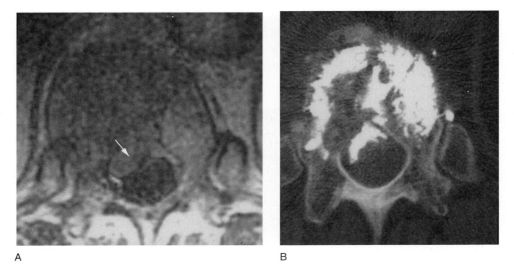

A   B

Figure 8-2. Partial destruction of the posterior wall with anterior epidural involvement by the tumor. (A) Axial MR image before PV. (B) Axial CT scan after PV. Note the cement in the epidural component of the tumor; there were no neurological complications. Both the "normal" and osteolytic parts of the vertebral body were injected.

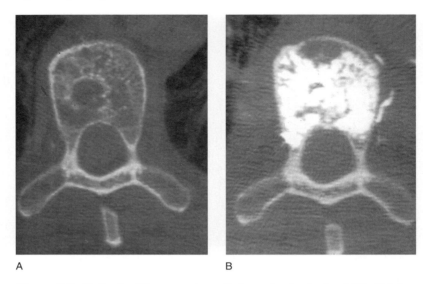

A   B

Figure 8-3. Patient with asymptomatic breast osteolysis of T8. (A) Axial CT before PV. (B) Axial CT after PV, which was performed because the extensive tumor placed the vertebral body at high risk for collapse.

The presence of multiple spinal lesions with diffuse back pain is not an indication for PV. However, PV for focal pain with multiple lesions is appropriate, but the treatment of several lesions may be required to give adequate pain relief (Fig. 8-4). The decision of which vertebra to treat depends on the correlation be-

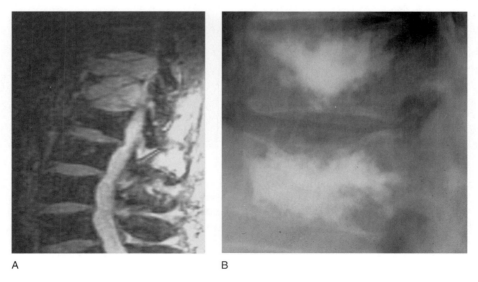

A   B

Figure 8-4. This patient presented with severe and focal back pain related to two metastatic lesions of T11–T12. (A) MR image and (B) lateral view after PV at two levels.

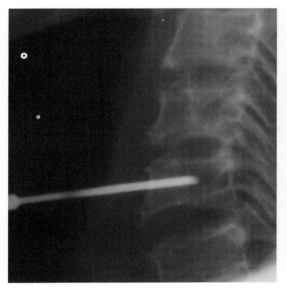
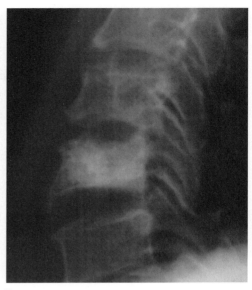

A   B

Figure 8-5. This patient presented with severe cervical pain related to a C5 lung cancer metastatic lesion. Lateral views before (A) and after (B) the injection of cement.

tween the imaging examination and physical findings. No more than three vertebrae should be treated at one session.

Although lesions in the thoracic and lumbar spine are often treated with PV, those in the cervical region can be treated operatively without major surgical exposure. However, based on the situation, patient's condition, and age, PV may be useful for treating cervical metastatic lesions (Fig. 8-5). As in all levels of the spine, metastatic lesions are associated with a high risk of epidural invasion or spinal cord damage in the presence of posterior wall compromise.

Contraindications to PV with spinal metastatic lesions include (1) complete collapse of the vertebra (generally there needs to be 25–30% of the original height remaining to allow successful PV[12]), (2) osteoblastic lesions (unless there is a mixed sclerotic and destructive lesion with focal pain and collapse) (Fig. 8-6), (3) nerve root or spinal cord compression and/or epidural or foraminal extension of the tumor, (4) diffuse (nonfocal) back pain, (5) complete destruction of the vertebra, or (6) coagulation disorders (platelets < 100,000, prothrombin time > 3 above the upper limits of normal, and partial thromboplastin time > 1.5 times normal).

Patient Selection and Evaluation

Generally, patients are referred for three main reasons: known cancer and back pain related to a spinal metastasis, known can-

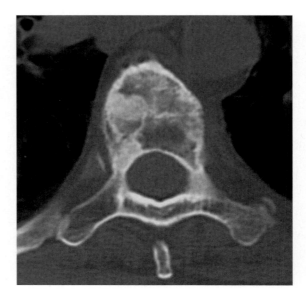

Figure 8-6. Breast metastatic and mixed osteolytic and osteoblastic lesions at T9 in a patient presenting with severe back pain.

cer and a recently diagnosed but asymptomatic spinal lesion, or back pain and suspicious lesions but no known diagnosis. Patient evaluations should consider all available clinical information. The clinical examination should identify the focal pain that correlates to the lesion considered for PV. The pain usually increases when the patient is standing and decreases when the patient is recumbent. The patient's pain should be severe, altering activities of daily living or requiring substantial use of analgesics. This pain should be documented with measurement instruments such as a visual analog scale or a quality-of-life questionnaire.

The pain described by the patient and detected on the clinical examination should be compared with the findings on plain radiographs, magnetic resonance (MR) imaging, and computed tomography (CT) and nuclear medicine scans. These diagnostic studies should be assessed for osteolysis, the degree of collapse, extension of tumor into the epidural space, and compression of neural tissue. It is difficult to predict future collapse associated with vertebral destruction, but the CT scan is best for detecting destruction of the posterior vertebral wall and determining whether the lesion is osteoblastic or osteolytic. Usually 50% or more of the vertebra needs to be destroyed before there is substantial risk of collapse (Fig. 8-3).

Once the patient has been found to meet the criteria indicating a need for PV, the procedure should be completely discussed with the patient and his or her family. This discussion should include the potential benefits of PV, its palliative nature, and the risks associated with the procedure. Finally, the patient should undergo a preanesthetic evaluation, electrocardiogram (ECG), and laboratory screen (complete blood cell count/platelets, electrolytes, prothrombin time/partial thromboplastin time, blood urea nitrogen/creatinine).

Technique

The technique for PV of malignant lesions is the same as that used for other indications (see Chapter 6). When the primary cancer is not known or if there is doubt about the cause of the vertebral lesion, a biopsy should precede the vertebroplasty. The cannula placed for cement injection will accommodate a 15- to 18-gauge biopsy device. These two procedures can be performed in one session because the presence of malignancy does not preclude PV.

To obtain good structural reinforcement of a partially destroyed vertebral body, both the destroyed and normal parts of the vertebra should be filled (Figs. 8-1 and 8-2).[11] Therefore, a bilateral transpedicular approach is usually required to achieve maximal filling of malignant lesions.

The distribution of cement must be monitored in real time with a high-quality fluoroscope. It is most important to examine the lateral view because this projection reveals leaks that occur laterally. Cement injections should be stopped immediately when the cement approaches the posterior vertebral wall. It is not important that the fill be homogeneous in distribution. A partial fill of the vertebral body can provide good pain relief. Pain relief has not been shown to be related to the quantity of cement injected.[12,13] However, if too little cement is injected, there remains the possibility of additional vertebral compression with weight bearing. Belkoff et al.[14] have shown in vitro that 4 to 6 mL of cement are needed to restore initial strength to osteoporotic vertebra (without osteolytic destruction). This study provides an approximation of the minimal volume that may be desired for structural reinforcement.

Our standard needle size varies from 10 to 13 gauge for the lumbar and thoracic spine. A 15-gauge needle is usually used in the cervical area. Smaller gauge needles have been used with a more liquid cement mix.[15–17] Although we think this technique is associated with a higher risk of cement leak and with resultant clinical complications, an interesting technical approach might be to use several needles inserted into the osteolytic lesion, with small amounts of cement injected via each needle.

Results

In 1989 Lapras et al.[15] were the first to report the use of PV for an L1 metastatic lesion. This early experience was encouraging because the patient experienced good pain relief and was able to resume walking. This report was followed by Kaemmerlen et al., who found that 80% of 20 patients experienced substantial pain relief from PV for malignant lesions within 48 h.[16] In 1996 Weill et al.[12] found that more than 75% of the patients in their series experienced pain relief and improved quality of life after PV. The results were durable for 6 months or longer in 73% of the patients. Finally, Cortet et al.[18] reported a 97% positive response rate for patients with malignant lesions within 48 h after PV. The pain relief was complete in 13.5% and substantially improved in 55%. The remaining 30% of the patients rated their improvement as moderate. The improvement was durable and unchanged in 75% at more than 6 months. Nevertheless, although substantial, the quality and quantity of pain relief after PV for malignant lesions appears to be less than that found in osteoporotic lesions treated with PV.

The mechanisms of pain relief in patients with malignant lesions are still not completely known. Stabilization of microfractures and reduction of mechanical forces are certainly the main factors. Tumor ischemia induced by the injection of cement into a solid lesion may also play a role. Destruction of the nerve endings in response to chemical (cytotoxic effect of the monomer) and thermal (exothermic reaction of the cement) forces has been postulated, but these mechanisms likely play a relatively minor role.[19] The necrotizing effect of the cement on the tumor mass may extend for a short distance beyond the limits of the margins of the polymethylmethacrylate (PMMA)[20] and may be a factor in the low rate of recurrence at the site of the PV even without complementary treatments.

Side Effects and Complications

A more complete description of the potential complications associated with PV is provided in Chapter 10. It is known that the incidence of cement leaks with PV for malignant lesions is much higher than that associated with osteoporotic fractures. This fact is almost surely attributable to the cortical destruction associated with the malignant lesions. The incidence of transient and persistent radiculopathy after PV for malignant disease is between 5 and 10%.[11–13,21] Our personal experience with the most recent 200 patients is a 5% complication rate; most of such complications are transient.

Problems that create pain may be transient and amenable to therapy with nonsteroidal antiinflammatory medications or local steroid injections. Radiculopathy may require surgical intervention to remove cement that might be producing a compressive effect on nerve roots (Fig. 8-7). The level of intervention is dictated by the patient's complaints. Minor pain should be

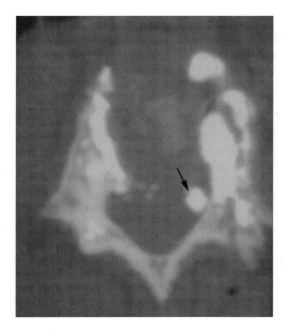

Figure 8-7. L4 breast cancer osteolytic metastatic lesion. Cement leaked into the radicular canal (arrow), inducing severe radiculopathy that resolved after surgical removal of the extravasated cement.

treated nonoperatively, whereas all motor dysfunction warrants an immediate surgical consultation. Any side effect (mild or major) should prompt reexamination to determine the explanation. Usually a CT scan is the most direct study for identifying a cement leak.

Percutaneous Vertebroplasty and Other Therapies

Radiation therapy alone can give partial or complete pain relief in 75 to 90% of patients.[22,23] However, this analgesic effect is obtained only after a delay of 10 to 20 days, and there is little strengthening of the vertebra, which leaves the vertebra at long-term risk for additional collapse and pain. Because PV does not diminish the positive effects of radiation (tumor elimination in the radiated field),[24] we believe that PV and radiation should be considered to be complementary therapies. Percutaneous vertebroplasty can be used to obtain rapid pain relief and to offer reinforcement to the involved vertebra. Radiation should help reduce local tumor recurrence.

When there are clinical signs of nerve or cord compression in patients with spinal metastases presenting with neurological symptoms, surgery is usually indicated. These procedures can be very complex and may require both anterior and posterior approaches to accomplish corporectomy and place instrumentation for spinal stabilization.[25] Analysis of vertebral involvement may occasionally indicate that appropriate use of PV can reduce the amount of surgery needed. Percutaneous reinforcement of involved vertebra may eliminate the need for an anterior approach in some patients.[11,12] With the anterior column support provided by PV, a posterior approach can be used for laminectomy to decompress the spine and stabilize it with posterior instrumentation. In patients with a shortened life span, this less invasive procedure should provide palliative improvement and a shorter period of convalescence.

The main concern when planning PV and chemotherapy is the effect of the chemotherapy on platelets, coagulation factors, and immunization. When possible, PV should precede chemotherapy.

Other local percutaneous therapies for metastatic lesions may be used. Thermal ablation or direct injection of absolute ethanol may be used for small lesions.[26] Intraarterial embolization may be used for large and hypervascularized tumors.[27] Percutaneous vertebroplasy must be used or combined with these treatments if structural reinforcement is to be achieved.

Part II: Multiple Myeloma

Anne Cotten, Nathalie Boutry, and Bernard Cortet

Pathology and Patient Demographics

Multiple myeloma is a monoclonal proliferation of malignant plasma cells that usually affects the bone marrow.[28] The peak incidence occurs during the sixth decade of life. The median survival time is 3 years. This disease is slightly more common in men than in women and affects three in 100,000 persons annually.[28]

Excessive bone resorption due to an increase of proinflammatory cytokines is a characteristic feature of the disease.[29-31] Diffuse osteoporosis and focal osteolytic lesions are thought to be potential causes of fractures in patients with multiple myeloma, and such fractures most frequently involve the spine.[32-34] Indeed, vertebral compression fractures are present in 55 to 70% of patients with multiple myeloma and represent the initial clinical sign in 34 to 64% of such patients.[35-38] Despite major improvements in chemotherapy, bone pain and widespread vertebral collapses are responsible for disability, respiratory restriction, and (sometimes) neurological complications.[39] All these conditions decrease the quality of life in patients with multiple myeloma.

In approximatively 5% of patients with plasma cell myeloma, solitary bone plasmocytoma represents the only disease feature. The diagnosis requires histological evidence of a monoclonal plasma cell infiltrate in one bone lesion, absence of other bone lesions on skeletal radiographs, and lack of marrow plasmacytosis elsewhere.[40] Two thirds of such patients develop multiple myeloma within 3 years after the discovery of a plasmacytoma; one third have no tumor progression for more than 10 years after discovery.[40–45] Early progression most likely results from occult generalized disease that was not recognized at diagnosis. Magnetic resonance imaging, more sensitive than conventional radiography for the detection of myeloma lesions, may indicate additional foci that represent occult myeloma.[40]

Technique

The procedure (guidance for needle positioning, needle route, etc.) in myelomatous vertebral lesions is not substantially different from that for other indications.[5,12,46,47] The transpedicular approach, when possible, is preferred. However, it should be remembered that the distribution of cement and the risk of cement leaks depend on the radiological appearance of the vertebral lesions.

Most of the vertebral collapses in patients with myeloma appear benign on radiographs and MR imaging, with a distribution similar to that observed in osteoporotic fractures.[30] When PV is performed for such collapses, the distribution of PMMA is frequently homogeneous in the vertebral body, and a single injec-

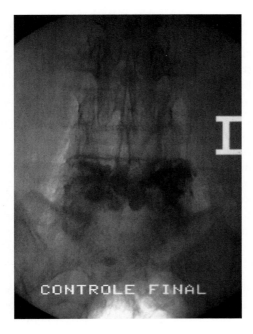

Figure 8-8. Homogeneous distribution of PMMA in the vertebral body of L5.

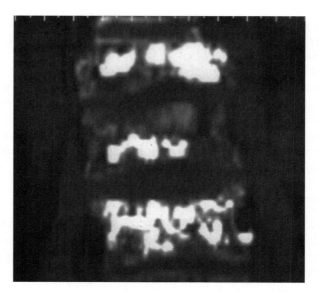

Figure 8-9. Three examples of inhomogeneous cement fill that may occur in myelomatous vertebral bodies.

tion of cement may be sufficient (Fig. 8-8). The risk of leaks of cement is small, especially if a cement more viscous than that normally used for PV is injected. Venous leaks are commonly observed if cement with a liquid consistency is injected in such lesions.[13]

When a lytic destructive lesion is demonstrated on conventional radiographs or CT scan, the degree of lesion filling is more varied and the risk of cement leakage is higher, possibly because of the different texture of this type of lesion. However, the distribution of cement obtained is usually better than that in osteolytic metastases (Fig 8-9).

Solitary bone plasmocytoma frequently appears as an osteolytic but trabeculated lesion[48] with cortical osteolysis frequently present, but only in some places (Fig. 8-10). The quality of the distribution of cement usually is intermediate between the two types of vertebral lesion demonstrated in multiple myeloma as just described.

Results

As in metastases and osteoporotic vertebral collapses, pain relief after PV for myeloma occurs within hours or days (usually within 24 h) after the procedure, sometimes after a transient worsening of pain. More than 70% of patients with multiple myeloma experience marked or complete pain relief.[5,12,13,46,47]

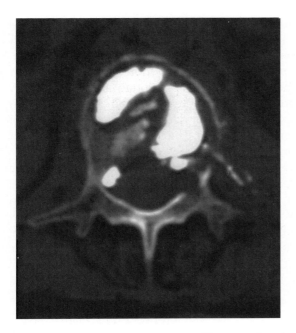

Figure 8-10. Solitary bone plasmocytoma: CT scan showing a small epidural leak.

Percutaneous Vertebroplasty and Other Therapies

Vertebrectomy is rarely performed in patients with myeloma because of the multifocal nature of the disease, but radiation therapy, in association with chemotherapy, has a major role in the management of such patients. Even so, this combination therapy does not address several treatment issues completely. First, its rapid and highly effective therapeutic effect on epidural involvement and neurological compression is well documented, and it is of great importance for patients at risk for spinal cord compression, which occurs in 10 to 15% of patients.[49] Second, local radiation therapy is effective for solitary bone plasmocytoma because it may prevent tumor growth. However, patients with multiple marrow lesions respond less satisfactorily to local radiation therapy than do the patients with a single lesion, and either type of local tumor may recur. Third, radiation therapy has been associated with a reduced incidence of vertebral fractures and focal marrow lesions[50] and with bone healing, remodeling, and reossification resulting in local reinforcement.[51] However, the bone reconstruction is minimal and delayed (2–4 months after the start of irradiation) and sometimes is preceded by transitory osteoporosis, which increases the risk of vertebral collapse and consequently of neural compression. Finally, radiation therapy usually results in partial or complete pain relief, with most patients experiencing some relief within 10 to 14 days. However some patients (5–10%) may experience insufficient pain relief and may be unable to tolerate additional radiation therapy.

Therefore, PV has an interesting place in the management of focal complicated myeloma lesions: it may provide rapid pain relief and vertebral stabilization when the lesion threatens the stability of the spine. Because such vertebral lesions are of clinical importance to the quality of life of patients with myeloma, PV may prevent a part of the morbidity and some of the mortality associated with the disease.[39] However, because in this clinical setting PV is a palliative procedure that does not prevent tumor growth, whenever possible it should be used in conjunction with radiation and chemotherapy for patients with myeloma.

Part III: Benign Tumors

Hervé Deramond, Anne Cotten,
and Claude Depriester

Pathology and Patient Demographics

Vertebral hemangiomas are common abnormalities. They have been found in 10% of spines at autopsy[52] or incidentally discovered on imaging studies. In rare cases, they can be aggressive lesions in terms of clinical and/or radiographic findings.

From a clinical point of view, aggressive VHs can be differentiated as painful VHs and VHs with neurological symptoms. The most frequent symptom is severe, mechanical back pain that increases with movement, even minimal movement such as shifting position in a chair. The tumor's progression is associated with a deterioration in the quality of life. Neurological signs can be related to nerve root and/or spinal cord compression by the VH invading the neural foramina or the epidural space. These neurologic signs can be acute or progressive.

From a radiological point of view, nonaggressive VHs can be diagnosed on plain films, CT scan, and/or MR imaging studies. Plain radiographs show localized and regular vertical striation of the vertebral body affected by the VH (Fig. 8-11A). The diagnostic CT scan shows a loss of the trabecular bone and thickening of the remaining vertical osseous network. The hypodense areas that appear surrounding the trabeculae on CT are fatty tissue that has replaced degenerated VH (Fig. 8-11B). The fatty component could be evidence of the nonprogressive nature of that part of the lesion.[53] Magnetic resonance imaging shows a typical hypersignal on T1-weighted images induced by the fatty stroma of the lesion (Fig. 8-11C). All these modalities show a well-

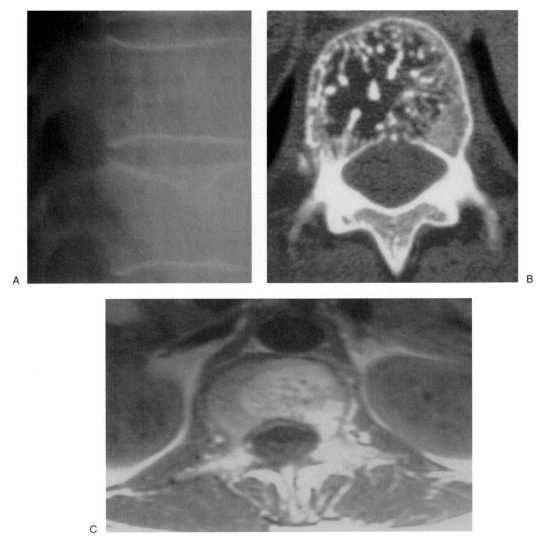

Figure 8-11. Nonaggressive VH. (A) Lateral radiograph showing localized and regular vertical striation of the vertebral body. (B) Axial CT scan showing loss of the trabecular bone and thickening of the remaining vertical osseous network, containing predominantly fatty stroma. (C) Axial T1-weighted MR image showing high signal intensity stroma related to fatty degeneration of a VH.

demarcated lesion in part or all of the vertebral body, without involvement of the cortical bone. Most of these lesions (which can occur singly or at multiple levels) are asymptomatic and are discovered only incidentally.

Radiologically aggressive VHs are characterized by the involvement of the whole vertebral body, locationed (frequently) in the thoracic area, an irregular honeycomb appearance of trabeculation, an expanded and poorly defined cortical bone, and swelling of the soft tissues.[54] On CT (Fig. 8-12A) and MR images (Fig. 8-12B), there is little or none of the fatty component usually seen with nonaggressive VHs. Imaging via CT and MR provides the best delineation of the extension of the VH to the paravertebral tissues. The epidural extension is best seen after intravenous injection of contrast (Fig. 8-12C). This epidural involvement can induce spinal cord and/or nerve root compression. Frequently VH extends to the posterior neural arch, involving the whole vertebra (Fig. 8-12A).

Other signs of an aggressive VH include an increase in the size of the VH on two successive radiographic examinations; expansion of the cortical bone, or a periosteal osseous formation that induces a spinal canal stenosis; and a weakened vertebral body and possible vertebral collapse occurring spontaneously or secondary to low-energy trauma (Fig. 8-13).

In most cases, VHs with radiographic signs of aggressiveness are symptomatic. Aggressive VHs can occur (singly or at multiple levels) in combination with the nonaggressive form.

Classification and Indications

Vertebral hemangiomas can be classified into one of four groups depending on their clinical and radiographic manifestations[47]: (1) asymptomatic VH without radiographic signs of aggressiveness (incidental discovery), (2) symptomatic (i.e, severe back pain) VH without radiographic signs of aggressiveness, (3) asymptomatic VH with radiographic signs of aggressiveness (incidental discovery), and (4) symptomatic VH with radiographic signs of aggressiveness. Group 4 can be divided into two subgroups: (a) VH with epidural extension and (b) VH without epidural extension but inducing severe back pain.

There are no indications for PV treatment for patients in group 1. For patients in group 2, PV is indicated because of severe back pain related to a VH even in the absence of radiographic signs of aggressiveness. The indication is easier to confirm in the thoracic region when there is only an isolated VH to explain the back pain. It is often difficult to appreciate the role of such a VH in the cervical area and even more so at the lumbar level, where associated degenerative disorders can induce the same pain.

Patients in group 3 require close monitoring with annual clinical and MR imaging examinations for progression of the VH. Percutaneous vertebroplasty is indicated only in patients for whom regular, long-term follow-up is not possible or for whom the VH becomes symptomatic or presents an evolution on successive radiographic studies.

Percutaneous vertebroplasty is indicated for all patients in group 4: the technique will vary depending on the progressive

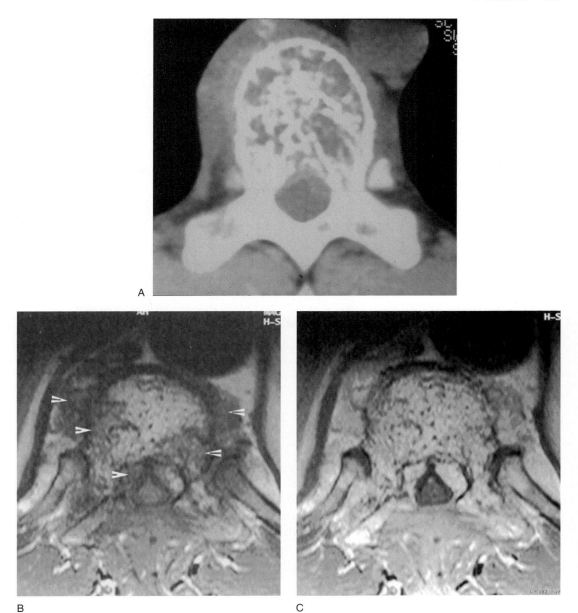

Figure 8-12. Aggressive VH. (A) Axial CT scan showing involvement of the whole vertebra with epidural and paravertebral extension. (B) Axial T1-weighted MR image showing epidural and paravertebral extension. The progressive parts of the lesion appear as an isosignal on noncontrast images (arrowheads). (C) Contrast-enhanced axial T1-weighted MR image showing hyperdense signal of the highly vascularized lesion.

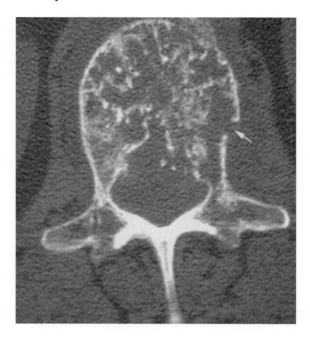

Figure 8-13. Aggressive VH. This axial CT scan of a patient presenting with severe back pain after falling on her back showed a VCF.

nature and severity of the neurological signs. Patients with an acute myelopathy or cauda equina syndrome should be treated by a combination of PV and surgery, as discussed later in the section entitled Technique. Patients presenting with progressive neurological signs should be treated with PV and percutaneous injection of absolute ethanol (see Technique). In a symptomatic patient with an aggressive VH but without epidural extension, PV alone is the treatment of choice.

Patient Evaluation

In general, patients present for evaluation for one of three reasons: incidental imaging diagnosis of an asymptomatic VH, severe back pain related to a VH, or neurological signs related to a VH. Evaluation of the patient should include all available clinical information. The clinical examination should elucidate focal pain or neurological signs that correlate with the lesion to be considered for PV. Pain should be documented with measurement instruments such as a visual analog scale or quality-of-life questionnaires (e.g., SF-36).[55]

The pain described by the patient and detected on the clinical examination should be compared with the findings on plain radiographs, MR imaging, and CT. At the lumbar and cervical levels, particularly in patients with radiographically nonaggressive VH, the clinician should attempt to confirm the relationship between the pain and the VH: that is, for PV to be indicated, degenerative lesions should be excluded as the possible origin of the pain. The MR images and CT scans should be assessed to differentiate between aggressive and nonaggressive VH, to determine any extension of the VH into the epidural space and neural foramina, and to evaluate for compression of neural tissue.

Once the criteria for PV have been met, the procedure should be completely discussed with the patient and his or her family. The discussion should include the potential benefits of PV and the risks associated with the procedure. Finally, the patient should undergo a preanesthetic evaluation, ECG, and laboratory screen (complete blood count/platelets, electrolytes, prothrombin time, partial thromboplastin time, blood urea nitrogen/creatinine).

Technique

According to the clinical presentation and radiographic signs, PV can be performed by using acrylic cement alone or with a combined treatment of acrylic cement followed by injection of glue or absolute ethanol.[3,47,56,57]

Percutaneous Vertebroplasty
When a VH presents without epidural involvement in patients complaining of pain, the treatment goals are to fill the defect (Fig. 8-14), obtain a structural reinforcement of the vertebral body, and provide pain relief. The needle must be inserted into the anterior part of the VH by a transpedicular approach. If the VH involves only a part of the vertebral body, it is possible to fill the whole malformation with only one injection and a single puncture (Fig. 8-15). If the whole vertebral body is involved, a bilateral transpedicular approach is usually required to fill the lesion.

Percutaneous Vertebroplasty with Complementary Injection of Ethanol
When a VH invades the anterior epidural space with no or only minor neurological symptoms, a complementary injection of absolute ethanol may be used to sclerose the lesion completely. This procedure is accomplished in four steps. First, the affected vertebral body is injected with acrylic cement via a unilateral or bilateral transpedicular approach. Second, a site is found around or in the vertebral body that has not been injected with cement, and an 18-gauge needle is inserted into it (Fig. 8-16). Third, the potential distribution of the sclerosing agent is checked by slowly injecting 1 to 4 mL of contrast medium; the quantity needed to inject the epidural component is noted and defines the amount

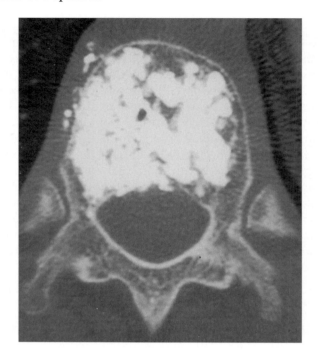

Figure 8-14. Axial CT scan after an injection of acrylic cement into a VH.

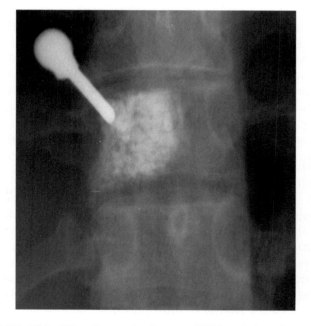

Figure 8-15. This AP radiograph shows a VH involving three quarters of the vertebral body, which was filled with acrylic cement; a unilateral transpedicular approach was used.

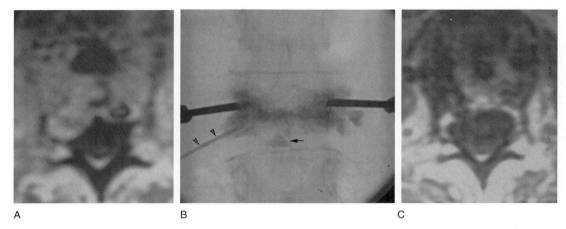

A   B   C

Figure 8-16. This patient had an aggressive VH with an epidural component. (A) Preoperative T1-weighted MR image. (B) AP view showing injection of the vertebral body part of the VH with acrylic cement. An 18-gauge needle was inserted into a part of the vertebral body that was not injected with cement (arrowheads), and alcohol was injected into the remaining part of the VH. Note the leakage of cement into the adjacent disks (arrow). (C) Resolution of the epidural VH 3 months after PV.

to be used for the subsequent injection of ethanol. Fourth, the absolute ethanol, usually no more than 4 mL, is slowly injected. If the VH involves the posterior neural arch, it is possible in the same procedure to use one or several needles to puncture that component and to obtain a complete sclerosis of the malformation, injecting no more than 1 mL of ethanol by each needle.

Heiss et al.[58] were the first to report the use of absolute ethanol ($\leq$ 50 mL) for the sclerosis of aggressive VH. However, they did not use an accompanying injection of acrylic cement. Two years later, they reported that two of seven patients had additional VCFs, presumably related to focal vertebral osteonecrosis secondary to the injection of a large amount of ethanol (40 and 50 mL, respectively).[59] Using PV before the injection of ethanol prevents such a complication by providing structural reinforcement of the vertebral body and by decreasing the amount of alcohol needed for sclerosing the VH (no more than 4 mL in our experience).

Percutaneous Vertebroplasty with Complementary Injection of Glue

In the presence of VH associated with an epidural component and acute clinical signs of compression of the spinal cord or cauda equina, the goal of PV is to reinforce the vertebral body and to make laminectomy and surgical excision of the epidural hemangioma easier by completely devascularizing the VH. This goal is accomplished by combining a PV procedure accompanied by an injection of *N*-butyl cyanoacrylate glue (opacified) on day 1 and surgery on day 2.[47,57]

The PV-with-glue procedure has five steps. First, the vertebral body invaded by the VH (Fig. 8-17A) is injected with acrylic cement via a unilateral or bilateral transpedicular approach. Second, an 18-gauge needle is inserted into the remaining VH that has not been injected with acrylic cement (Fig. 8-17B). Third, the predictable distribution of the glue is checked by the slow injection of up to 4 mL of contrast medium. Fourth, after the needle has been carefully washed with a nonionic solution (glucose serum) to avoid the early polymerization of the glue in the needle, 3 to 5 mL of the glue mixture is slowly injected under fluoroscopic control to fill the compressive epidural component of the lesion (Fig. 8-17C). Fifth (if necessary), the percutaneous embolization of the remaining component of the VH is completed by injecting glue via one or several needles inserted into the posterior neural arch (Fig. 8-17D, E). Laminectomy and surgical excision of the epidural component of the VH (simplified by the PV) usually are planned for the following day (Fig. 8-17F).

With our experience of four such patients, we think it might be possible to avoid surgery by using the PV-with-ethanol procedure. Even patients with acute neurological signs showed no worsening clinical signs after such a PV procedure. Thus, using a sclerosing agent could allow a progressive and complete improvement of the neurologic signs and avoid the need for surgery.[59]

Using Computed Tomography for Percutaneous Vertebroplasty
Gangi et al.[60] described the technique for PV using CT: the needle is placed precisely and safely under CT guidance, and the injection of the cement is performed under real-time fluoroscopic control. Most of the time, a good biplane fluoroscopy unit allows a fast and safe procedure for PV. However, when a complementary injection of absolute ethanol or glue is needed for the treatment of VHs, checking the distribution of the acrylic cement into the vertebral body and setting the 18-gauge needle into a part of the vertebral body not injected with cement or into the posterior neural arch requires the use of CT (Fig. 8-17B).

Results

In the first published cases, PV was used to treat VHs.[3,47] Of those first 11 patients, 10 had complete relief of pain after the PV procedure. The literature documents substantial pain reduction in more than 80% of patients whose VHs were treated by PV.[47,58,61,62]

Deramond et al.[47] have treated 61 patients with symptomatic VH. With a long-term follow-up (≤ 15 years), structural reinforcement was obtained in all patients, there was no change in

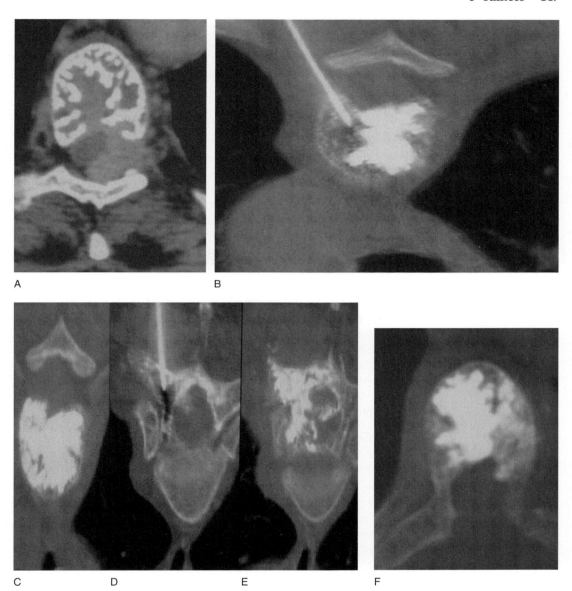

Figure 8-17. This patient presented with an acute spinal cord compression related to an aggressive thoracic VH. (A) Axial CT scan before PV. (B) An axial CT scan of the injection of acrylic cement into three quarters of the vertebral body part affected by the VH. Under CT guidance, an 18-gauge needle was inserted into the portion of the vertebral body lesion not injected with cement. (C) Axial CT scan showing the distribution of glue in the remaining part of the vertebral body but without injection of the epidural component. (D) Axial CT scan showing the insertion under CT guidance of an 18-gauge needle into the posterior neural arch invaded by the VH. (E) Axial CT scan showing the distribution of the glue into the posterior neural arch and the epidural component of the VH. (F) Axial CT scan after surgical laminectomy and excision of the epidural VH.

the shape of the vertebral body, and relief of severe back pain was obtained for more than 90% of the patients. Only once did evolution of the epidural part of the VH occur. In that case, PV was conducted at the C2 level and acrylic cement alone (with no sclerosing agent) was injected into the vertebral body. Early results were good, but after 3 years the epidural component suddenly increased, and the growth continued despite radiation therapy. The patient died 4 years later from neurological complications.[56]

A review of the results in terms of the classification groups described earlier shows the following: group 2 (38 patients; treated with PV), complete pain relief in more than 90% (35 patients), with no recurrence of the lesion; group 4a-i (12 patients; all treated with PV, five also treated with ethanol injection), all had cessation of progressive neurologic signs, no evolution (3–7 years of follow-up) or recurrence of the epidural component (except for the first patient already described), and the epidural component disappeared in two of the five treated with ethanol; group 4a-ii (four patients; treated with PV, glue, and laminectomy), no evolution (3–7 years of follow-up) or recurrence of epidural component, and disappearance of acute neurological signs; group 4b (seven patients; treated with PV), complete relief of back pain in all patients and no change in the lesion.

Side Effects and Complications

In the first group of 54 patients with VH treated by PV, there were only two complications: both were intercostal neuralgias that healed after local injection with steroids and anesthetic.[47] These complications were related to leakage of cement into foraminal veins and occurred among the first patients treated. One patient had been injected with a cement having a low radiopacity; the method was subsequently improved by adding tantalum powder.[56] In the second patient, intercostal neuralgia was related to a leakage of cement along the track of a needle inserted via an intercostal posterolateral approach (Craig technique),[63] which irritated the adjacent nerve root. The transpedicular approach avoids this complication.

Percutaneous Vertebroplasty and Other Therapies

Radiation Therapy

Radiation therapy alone with fractionated doses under 4000 cGy has been used to treat VH.[64,65] The risk of complication is low with these low doses, but the rate of recurrence is approximately 50%.[66] These considerations, combined with the efficacy of PV, have led us to believe that radiation therapy is no longer indicated for the treatment of VHs.

Laminectomy and Surgical Excision

Laminectomy and surgical excision of the epidural component of the lesion is the classical treatment for VH with neurological signs.[67,68] However, this surgery is often difficult because of the vascular nature of the lesion. In our experience, PV before surgery makes the excision easier and less risky. In addition, we think that in most patients with acute neurological signs, PV combined with ethanol injection may obviate surgery.

Transarterial Embolization

Transarterial embolization[69] provides excellent short-term results for aggressive VHs. However, evolution and recurrence of the VH is frequent. It is the classic treatment before surgery, with the goal of decreasing preoperative bleeding, but efficacy is variable. Moreover, transarterial embolization can be impossible or dangerous, with the risk of spinal cord infarction when a common artery supplies the VH and the spinal cord. In the early days of PV treatment, embolization was performed before PV,[56,57] but it quickly became evident that that procedure was unnecessary because PV provides a far more efficient in situ filling of the vascular malformation.

References

1. Parlier-Cuau C, Champsaur P, Nizard R, et al. Percutaneous removal of osteoid osteoma. *Radiol Clin North Am* 1998; 36(3):559–566.
2. Gladden ML, Jr, Gillingham BL, Hennrikus W, et al. Aneurysmal bone cyst of the first cervical vertebrae in a child treated with percutaneous intralesional injection of calcitonin and methylprednisolone. A case report. *Spine* 2000; 25(4):527–530.
3. Galibert P, Deramond H, Rosat P, et al. [Preliminary note on the treatment of vertebral angioma by percutaneous acrylic vertebroplasty.] *Neurochirurgie* 1987; 33(2):166–168.
4. Cardon T, Hachulla E, Flipo RM, et al. Percutaneous vertebroplasty with acrylic cement in the treatment of a Langerhans cell vertebral histiocytosis. *Clin Rheumatol* 1994; 13(3):518–521.
5. Cotten A, Boutry N, Cortet B, et al. Percutaneous vertebroplasty: state of the art. *Radiographics* 1998; 18(2):311–323.
6. Abrams HL, Spiro R, Goldstein N. Metastases in carcinoma. Analysis of 1000 autopsied cases. *Cancer* 1950; 3:74–85.
7. Malawer MM, Delandy TF. Treatment of metastatic cancer to bone. In: DeVita VT, Hellman S, Rosenberg SA, eds. *Cancer: Principles and Practice of Oncology.* 3rd ed. Philadelphia: JB Lippincott Co; 1989: 2298–2317.
8. Bontoux D, Azais I. Cancer secondaire des os. Clinique et epidémiologie. In: Bontoux D, Alcalay M, eds. *Cancer Secondaire des Os.* Paris: Expansion Scientifique Française; 1997:19–27.
9. Tubiana-Hulin M. Incidence, prevalence and distribution of bone metastases. *Bone* 1991; 12(suppl 1):S9–S10.
10. Tatsui H, Onomura T, Morishita S, et al. Survival rates of patients

with metastatic spinal cancer after scintigraphic detection of abnormal radioactive accumulation. *Spine* 1996; 21(18):2143–2148.

11. Deramond H, Depriester C, Toussaint P. [Vertebroplasty and percutaneous interventional radiology in bone metastases: techniques, indications, contra-indications.] *Bull Cancer Radiother* 1996; 83(4):277–282.

12. Weill A, Chiras J, Simon JM, et al. Spinal metastases: indications for and results of percutaneous injection of acrylic surgical cement. *Radiology* 1996; 199(1):241–247.

13. Cotten A, Dewatre F, Cortet B, et al. Percutaneous vertebroplasty for osteolytic metastases and myeloma: effects of the percentage of lesion filling and the leakage of methyl methacrylate at clinical follow-up. *Radiology* 1996; 200(2):525–530.

14. Belkoff SM, Mathis JM, Jasper LE, et al. The biomechanics of vertebroplasty: the effect of cement volume on mechanical behavior. *Spine* 2001; 26(14):1537–1541.

15. Lapras C, Mottolese C, Deruty R, et al. [Percutaneous injection of methylmethacrylate in osteoporosis and severe vertebral osteolysis (Galibert's technic).] *Ann Chir* 1989; 43(5):371–376.

16. Kaemmerlen P, Thiesse P, Bouvard H, et al. [Percutaneous vertebroplasty in the treatment of metastases. Technic and results.] *J Radiol* 1989; 70(10):557–562.

17. Kaemmerlen P, Thiesse P, Jonas P, et al. Percutaneous injection of orthopedic cement in metastatic vertebral lesions [letter]. *N Engl J Med* 1989; 321(2):121.

18. Cortet B, Cotten A, Boutry N, et al. Percutaneous vertebroplasty in patients with osteolytic metastases or multiple myeloma [see comments]. *Rev Rhum Engl Ed* 1997; 64(3):177–183.

19. Deramond H, Wright NT, Belkoff SM. Temperature elevation caused by bone cement polymerization during vertebroplasty. *Bone* 1999; 25(2 suppl):17S–21S.

20. San Millan RD, Burkhardt K, Jean B, et al. Pathology findings with acrylic implants. *Bone* 1999; 25(2 suppl):85S–90S.

21. Chiras J, Depriester C, Weill A, et al. [Percutaneous vertebral surgery. Technics and indications.] *J Neuroradiol* 1997; 24(1):45–59.

22. Shepherd S. Radiotherapy and the management of metastatic bone pain. *Clin Radiol* 1988; 39(5):547–550.

23. Salazar OM, Rubin P, Hendrickson FR, et al. Single-dose half-body irradiation for the palliation of multiple bone metastases from solid tumors: a preliminary report. *Int J Radiat Oncol Biol Phys* 1981; 7:773–781.

24. Murray JA, Bruels MC, Lindberg RD. Irradiation of polymethylmethacrylate. In vitro gamma radiation effect. *J Bone Joint Surg* 1974; 56A(2):311–312.

25. Riley LH, Frassica DA, Kostuik JP, et al. Metastatic disease to the spine: diagnosis and treatment. *Instr Course Lect* 2000; 49:471–477.

26. Gangi A, Guth S, Dietemann JL, et al. Interventional musculoskeletal procedures. *Radiographics* 2001; 21(2):520.

27. Meder JF, Reizine D, Chiras J, et al. Apport de l'arthériographie dans le diagnostic et le traitement des tumeurs du rachis. *Rachis* 1992; 4(4):215–218.

28. Longo DL. Plasma cell disorders. In: Wilson JD, Braunwald E, Isselbacher KJ, et al., eds. *Harrison's Principles of Internal Medicine.* 12th ed. New York: McGraw-Hill; 1991:1412–1416.

29. Bataille R, Chappard D, Klein B. Mechanisms of bone lesions in multiple myeloma. *Hematol Oncol Clin North Am* 1992; 6(2):285–295.

30. Lecouvet FE, Vande Berg BC, Maldague BE, et al. Vertebral compression fractures in multiple myeloma. Part I. Distribution and appearance at MR imaging [see comments]. *Radiology* 1997; 204(1):195–199.

31. Salmon SE, Cassady JR. Plasma cell neoplasms. In: DeVita VT, Hellman S, Rosenberg SA, eds. *Cancer: Principles and Practice of Oncology.* 4th ed. Philadelphia: JB Lippincott Co; 1993:1984–2025.

32. de Gramont A, Benitez O, Brissaud P, et al. Quantification of bone lytic lesions and prognosis in myelomatosis. *Scand J Haematol* 1985; 34(1):78–82.

33. Kanis JA, McCloskey EV. Disorders of calcium metabolism and their management. In: Malpas JS, Bergsagel DE, Kyle RA, eds. *Myeloma: Biology and Management.* New York: Oxford University Press; 1995: 375–396.

34. Kapadia SB. Multiple myeloma: a clinicopathologic study of 62 consecutively autopsied cases. *Medicine (Baltimore)* 1980; 59(5):380–392.

35. Kyle RA. Multiple myeloma: review of 869 cases. *Mayo Clin Proc* 1975; 50(1):29–40.

36. Carson CP, Ackerman LV, Maltby JD. Plasma cell myeloma: a clinical, pathologic, and roentgenologic review of 90 cases. *Am J Clin Pathol* 1955; 25:849–888.

37. Riccardi A, Gobbi PG, Ucci G, et al. Changing clinical presentation of multiple myeloma. *Eur J Cancer* 1991; 27(11):1401–1405.

38. Spiess JL, Adelstein DJ, Hines JD. Multiple myeloma presenting with spinal cord compression. *Oncology* 1988; 45(2):88–92.

39. Lecouvet FE, Malghem J, Michaux L, et al. Vertebral compression fractures in multiple myeloma. Part II. Assessment of fracture risk with MR imaging of spinal bone marrow [see comments]. *Radiology* 1997; 204(1):201–205.

40. Moulopoulos LA, Dimopoulos MA, Weber D, et al. Magnetic resonance imaging in the staging of solitary plasmacytoma of bone. *J Clin Oncol* 1993; 11(7):1311–1315.

41. Knowling MA, Harwood AR, Bergsagel DE. Comparison of extramedullary plasmacytomas with solitary and multiple plasma cell tumors of bone. *J Clin Oncol* 1983; 1(4):255–262.

42. Chak LY, Cox RS, Bostwick DG, et al. Solitary plasmacytoma of bone: treatment, progression, and survival. *J Clin Oncol* 1987; 5(11):1811–1815.

43. Frassica DA, Frassica FJ, Schray MF, et al. Solitary plasmacytoma of bone: Mayo Clinic experience. *Int J Radiat Oncol Biol Phys* 1989; 16(1): 43–48.

44. Dimopoulos MA, Goldstein J, Fuller L, et al. Curability of solitary bone plasmacytoma. *J Clin Oncol* 1992; 10(4):587–590.

45. Holland J, Trenkner DA, Wasserman TH, et al. Plasmacytoma. Treatment results and conversion to myeloma. *Cancer* 1992; 69(6):1513–1517.

46. Murphy KJ, Deramond H. Percutaneous vertebroplasty in benign and malignant disease. *Neuroimaging Clin North Am* 2000; 10(3):535–545.

47. Deramond H, Depriester C, Galibert P, et al. Percutaneous vertebroplasty with polymethyl methacrylate. Technique, indications, and results. *Radiol Clin North Am* 1998; 36(3):533–546.

48. Huvos AG. Multiple myeloma including solitary osseous myeloma. In: *Bone Tumors: Diagnosis, Treatment, and Prognosis.* Philadelphia: WB Saunders Co; 1992:653–676.

49. Plowman PN. Radiotherapy of myeloma. In: Malpas JS, Bergsagel DE, Kyle RA, eds. *Myeloma: Biology and Management.* New York: Oxford University Press; 1995:314–321.

50. Lecouvet F, Richard F, Vande Berg B, et al. Long-term effects of localized spinal radiation therapy on vertebral fractures and focal lesions appearance in patients with multiple myeloma. *Br J Haematol* 1997; 96(4):743–745.

51. Hoskin PJ. Radiotherapy in the management of bone pain. *Clin Orthop* 1995; 312:105–119.

52. Schmorl G, Junghanns H. *The Human Spine in Health and Disease* (Besemann ES, transl. and ed.). 2nd ed. New York: Grune & Stratton; 1971.

53. Laredo JD, Assouline E, Gelbert F, et al. Vertebral hemangiomas: fat content as a sign of aggressiveness. *Radiology* 1990; 177(2):467–472.

54. Laredo JD, Reizine D, Bard M, et al. Vertebral hemangiomas: radiologic evaluation. *Radiology* 1986; 161(1):183–189.

55. Ware JE, Jr., Snow KK, Kosinski M, et al. *SF-36 Health Survey. Manual and Interpretation Guide.* Boston: The Health Institute; 1993.

56. Deramond H, Darrason R, Galibert P. [Percutaneous vertebroplasty with acrylic cement in the treatment of aggressive spinal angiomas.] *Rachis* 1989; 1(2):143–153.

57. Cotten A, Deramond H, Cortet B, et al. Preoperative percutaneous injection of methyl methacrylate and N-butyl cyanoacrylate in vertebral hemangiomas. *Am J Neuroradiol* 1996; 17(1):137–142.

58. Heiss JD, Doppman JL, Oldfield EH. Brief report: relief of spinal cord compression from vertebral hemangioma by intralesional injection of absolute ethanol [see comments]. *N Engl J Med* 1994; 331(8):508–511.

59. Heiss JD, Doppman JL, Oldfield EH. Treatment of vertebral hemangioma by intralesional injection of absolute ethanol [letter; comment]. *N Engl J Med* 1996; 334(20):1340.

60. Gangi A, Kastler BA, Dietemann JL. Percutaneous vertebroplasty guided by a combination of CT and fluoroscopy. *Am J Neuroradiol* 1994; 15(1):83–86.

61. Ide C, Gangi A, Rimmelin A, et al. Vertebral haemangiomas with spinal cord compression: the place of preoperative percutaneous vertebroplasty with methyl methacrylate. *Neuroradiology* 1996; 38(6): 585–589.

62. Martin JB, Jean B, Sugiu K, et al. Vertebroplasty: clinical experience and follow-up results. *Bone* 1999; 25(2 suppl):11S–15S.

63. Craig FS. Vertebral-body biopsy. *J Bone Joint Surg* 1956; 38A(1):93–102.

64. Yang ZY, Zhang LJ, Chen ZX, et al. Hemangioma of the vertebral column. A report on twenty-three patients with special reference to functional recovery after radiation therapy. *Acta Radiol Oncol* 1985; 24(2):129–132.

65. Pavlovitch JM, Nguyen JP, Djindjian M, et al. Radiotherapy of compressive vertebral hemangiomas. *Neurochirurgie* 1989; 35:296–298.

66. Nguyen JP, Djindjian M, Pavlovitch JM, et al. Vertebral hemangiomas with neurologic symptoms. Treatment. Results of the "Société Française de Neuro-Chirurgie" series. *Neurochirurgie* 1989; 35: 299–303.

67. Nguyen JP, Djindjian M, Gaston A, et al. Vertebral hemangiomas presenting with neurologic symptoms. *Surg Neurol* 1987; 27(4):391–397.

68. Nguyen JP, Djindjian M, Badiane S. Vertebral hemangiomas with neurologic symptoms. Clinical presentation. Results of the "Société Française de Neurochirurgie" series. *Neurochirurgie* 1989; 35:270–274.

69. Picard L, Bracard S, Roland J, et al. [Embolization of vertebral hemangioma. Technic-indications-results.] Embolisation des hemangiomes vertebraux. Technique-indications-resultats. *Neurochirurgie* 1989; 35(5):289–293.

9

Extreme Vertebroplasty: Techniques for Treating Difficult Lesions

John D. Barr and John M. Mathis

For most patients, the standard techniques for performing percutaneous vertebroplasty (PV) work very well. However, for patients with malignant disease causing severe cortical destruction, the usual techniques may be associated with a high incidence of cement extravasation and complications. Osteoporotic patients presenting with very severe vertebral body compression also represent a treatment challenge. Modification of the usual techniques may provide an alternative that allows better treatment for patients of both these types.

Computed Tomography and Fluoroscopy

Percutaneous vertebroplasty is useful for the treatment of selected patients with pain due to vertebral column malignancies, particularly patients who are poor surgical candidates and those with limited anticipated survival. The procedure may be performed to provide analgesia or spinal stabilization, or both. With the traditional fluoroscopically guided technique, PV for neoplastic lesions results in more frequent complications than PV for osteoporotic vertebral compression fractures (VCFs).[1] Most complications associated with PV for neoplastic lesions are secondary to extravasation of cement through cortical bone destroyed by the tumor. When an osteolytic lesion breaches the cortical barrier to the spinal canal or neural foramen, the probability of symptomatic cement extravasation increases markedly.[2,3] The risk that even small cement extravasations will be symptomatic is increased in the presence of spinal canal compromise or when the treatment involves an upper thoracic or cervical vertebra. To reduce the risk of extravasation, it is imperative that a properly opacified cement[4] and high-quality imaging equipment be used.[5] Even so, fluoroscopy alone may not provide resolution sufficient to permit one to visualize small, potentially symptomatic cement extravasations. In such complex and high-risk cases—that is, when the posterior wall is disrupted (Fig. 9-1) or when upper thoracic and cervical vertebral bodies are involved—a procedure using combined computed tomography (CT) and fluoroscopic guidance may be useful.[6]

Gangi and colleagues[7] were the first to describe the use of a combination of CT and fluoroscopic guidance for PV of both VCFs and osteolytic neoplasms. This technique typically uses a CT scanner in combination with a portable C-arm angiography system.[6] The primary advantage of using CT with fluoroscopy is that the CT scanner provides images that allow the operating physician to assess the three-dimensional distribution of the injected cement in exquisite detail (Fig. 9-2). By noting the prox-

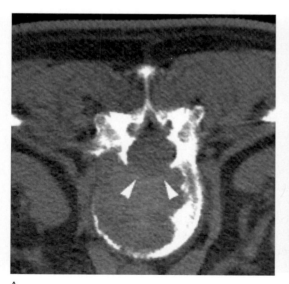 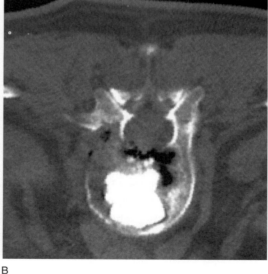

A   B

Figure 9-1. CT images of an L1 vertebra with trabecular and cortical destruction secondary to multiple myeloma. (A) Preoperative scan showing complete destruction of the posterior cortical wall (arrowheads). (B) Image after PV showing good filling of the anterior two thirds of the vertebral body. Note that air (which appears as dark areas posterior and lateral to the cement) was injected along with the cement during the procedure. The patient had relief of pain, and the vertebral body remained stable at 1-year follow-up.

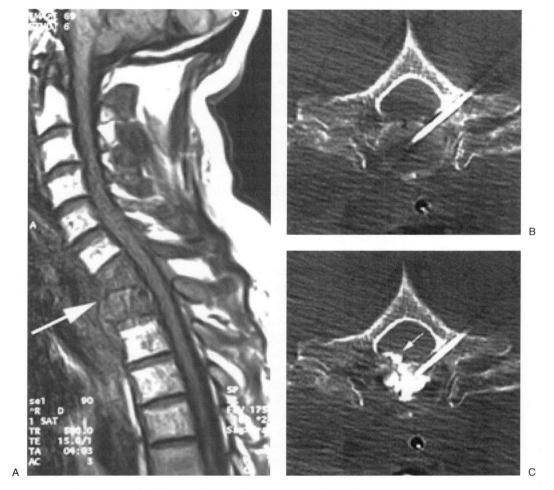

Figure 9-2. This patient's C7 and T1 vertebrae were infiltrated by a metastatic, mediastinal sarcoma. (A) Sagittal T1-weighted MR image showing tumor infiltration (arrow) at C7 and T1. The collapse of these vertebrae was associated with intractable pain. Visualization of this area fluoroscopically was nearly impossible because of shoulders. (B) CT image showing needle placed via a posterior transpedicular approach. (C) CT image during PV revealed a very small epidural leak of cement (arrow). The injection was terminated, and the patient had good pain relief without a clinical complication.

imity of the cement to the posterior vertebral margin (and epidural space), the operating physician can determine the need for, and safety of, injecting additional cement (Fig. 9-1). When treating the small upper thoracic vertebrae (Fig. 9-2)—areas that are commonly obscured by the shoulders on fluoroscopic images—the operating physician can obtain CT images showing the precise location of the needles for cement delivery. Similarly, the precise imaging capability of CT may be needed in the cervical spine because of the small size of the vertebra and because of the critical structures that must be avoided (i.e., cervical cord and carotid and vertebral vessels).

With combined CT and fluoroscopic imaging, either fluoroscopy or CT is used for the initial needle placement. When precise anatomic visualization is needed for needle placement (e.g., near the carotid artery), the patient is positioned in the CT scanner and CT guidance is used in placing the needle. Then the patient is removed from the scanner so that cement injection may begin under fluoroscopic monitoring. When precise visualization of cement is needed, the patient is transferred back into the scanner. If the injected cement is not in close proximity to the spinal canal or neural foramen, injection of very small quantities (0.1–0.2 mL) of cement may proceed under fluoroscopy with intermittent visualization using CT. This technique allows the injection of cement while maintaining a low probability of a clinically significant cement leak into the spinal canal or neural foramen.

However, there are several disadvantages to using the combined CT-fluoroscopy technique. Patients almost always need general anesthesia because most types of CT imaging are very sensitive to patient motion. Although transferring the patient in and out of the CT gantry can be done quickly with some practice, it is an added step and consumes time. Furthermore, when the patient is outside the scanner, the fluoroscope is limited to producing images in the lateral plane because of interference caused by the CT table on which the patient is positioned. The use of CT is also markedly more expensive than fluoroscopy alone. For these reasons, the use of CT is limited to the extraordinary (not routine) cases.

Notwithstanding the foregoing disadvantages, combined CT and fluoroscopy may help reduce the incidence of complications in difficult cases. For example, Barr et al.[6] reported on eight patients who underwent treatment for malignant lesions in 13 vertebrae. Four vertebrae (in three patients) without cortical destruction were treated with the usual fluoroscopically guided technique. Nine involved vertebrae in five patients who were treated by means of the modified technique using a combination of CT and fluoroscopic guidance. In four of those patients, eight vertebrae had posterior cortical disruption (Fig. 9-1). No symptomatic complications were observed in any of the patients so treated. Although these results are encouraging, the number of patients managed with combined CT and fluoroscopy is too small to establish efficacy of the procedure and does not allow us to make meaningful comparisons with using fluoroscopy alone.

An alternative to using combined CT and fluoroscopy is the use of CT-fluoroscopy (i.e., continuous CT), which allows real-time monitoring of the needle placement and cement injection.[8] Limitations of this technique include the difficulty of positioning the needle and performing the cement injection with the patient in the CT scanner. Injecting the cement while the patient is in a scanner causes the operating physician's hands to be exposed to the x-ray beam. If needle positioning and cement injection are prolonged, radiation doses to the physician and the patient may be undesirably high.

Coaxial Needle Placement and Exchange

Another technique that may be used when extremely precise cannula placement is needed is coaxial needle exchange. Coaxial needle exchange consists of using a small-diameter needle to serve as a guidewire for the subsequent placement of a large-diameter cannula for cement injection.[9] The small-diameter needle, typically a 20-gauge, 20-cm Chiba, is placed under fluoroscopic guidance. If combined CT and fluoroscopy is used, CT may be used to confirm good needle position before a large-bore cannula is introduced for cement injection. The Chiba needle can also be used to administer the local anesthetic for the subsequent PV procedure. Just before cannula placement, the hub of the needle is removed, and a small skin incision is made around the needle. The cannula of an 11-gauge needle is then advanced over the 20-gauge needle to the cortex. The 20-gauge needle, which served as a guidewire, is exchanged for the trocar of the 11-gauge needle. The 11-gauge needle (cannula and trocar) is then advanced into the vertebral body in the usual fashion.

Coaxial needle exchange is also helpful when cement extravasates before the vertebral body is adequately filled. For example, injected cement usually follows the path of least resistance. Therefore, it is not uncommon for cement to flow though a vertebral end plate fracture into the disk space, or through osteolytic defects in patients with neoplastic disease. Such extravasations, provided they are small, can serve a useful purpose. If injection is halted and the cement is allowed to polymerize, it will seal the cortical defects and prevent further extravasation of cement. Unfortunately, as the cement polymerizes, it will also occlude the cannula being used for the injection. This problem can be overcome by exchanging the cement-filled cannula for a new cannula so that more cement may be injected. To achieve an easy exchange, a 20-gauge Chiba needle is placed through the cement-filled cannula into the vertebral body. The cannula is then removed. Once the injected cement has polymerized, a new cannula is placed coaxially using the Chiba needle as a guidewire. The Chiba needle is then removed. The small-diameter Chiba needle has insufficient surface area for cement adherence, and it can be easily removed. Cement injection may then resume, the cement leaks having been effectively occluded by polymerized cement.

Fracture Instability and Height Restoration

Technically successful PV results in lasting analgesia for most patients. However, pain is not the only clinically significant problem caused by VCFs. Based on data from a prospective 8-year study of 9575 women, Kado and colleagues[10] reported a 23 to 34% increase in mortality for postmenopausal women with vertebral fractures (even if asymptomatic) relative to age-matched controls without fractures. Pulmonary disease, probably related to kyphosis, was the leading cause of death. Thus, restoration of vertebral height and the reduction or elimination of kyphosis are desirable therapeutic goals. Vertebral height restoration and reduction of kyphosis may be attained in some cases by using patient positioning or external traction. Barr et al.[11] noted that in some patients, there was fluoroscopically recognizable fracture instability that allowed some vertebral body height restoration with hyperextension or traction (Fig. 9-3). Thus, vertebral height

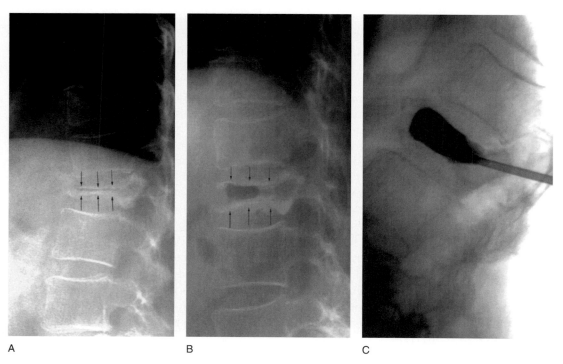

A   B   C

Figure 9-3. This patient had an extreme compression of T12 and continued severe pain 3 months after the fracture. (A) Lateral view showing the cortical margins of the compressed vertebra (arrows). The faint dark line centrally was created by a central vacuum phenomenon. (B) Traction was applied to the shoulder and legs, and lateral fluoroscopy revealed partial height restoration of the T12 collapse. The arrows highlight the cortical end plates. (C) Lateral fluoroscopic image during PV (after traction) shows cement filling the central cavity within the vertebra. The height restoration achieved with traction was maintained. The patient's pain resolved after PV, and her clinical status was stable at 9-month follow-up.

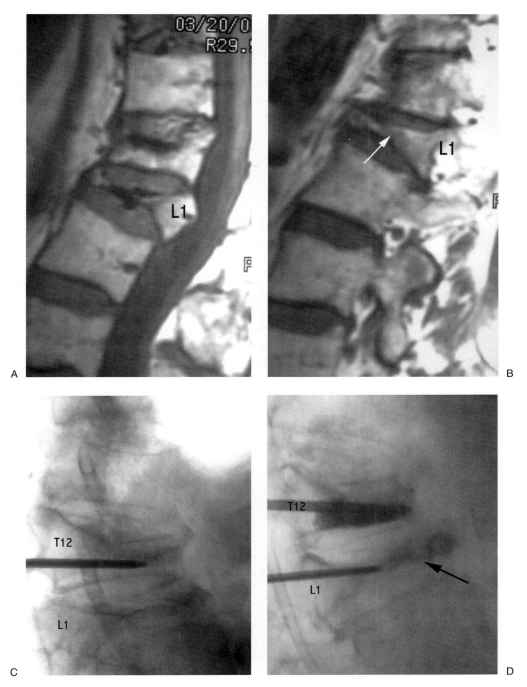

Figure 9-4. This patient had extreme compression of the L1 vertebra with less compression at T12. (A) A T1-weighted sagittal MR image (midline). (B) A more lateral MR image showing residual marrow space (arrow) in the L1 vertebra that might accept cement. Pain was localized to the area of T12-L1, so both vertebrae were treated with PV. (C) Lateral view after needle placement in T12 also showed the extreme compression of L1. (D) Lateral view after needle placement in L1 and early filling of the anterior L1 vertebra (arrow). A 13-gauge needle was used for L1 and an 11-gauge was used at T12. The patient experienced substantial pain relief from this two-level procedure.

loss and the resulting kyphosis may be a reversible effect of VCFs. Because of the generally frail structure of patients with osteoporosis, traction should be applied slowly and with the patient's cooperation to avoid injuries. Once vertebral body height has been regained and the patient is in hyperextension or in traction, the vertebral body can be injected with cement (Fig. 9-3). Experience with VCF reduction using traction is limited, but acute fractures appear to be more reducible because they have not had time to undergo early healing. Even so, one 8-month-old fracture presenting as a nonunion was successfully reduced by means of this technique.[11]

Treatment of Extreme Vertebral Collapse

In cases of extreme vertebral body collapse (i.e., > 70% loss of vertebral body height), PV is typically not used.[12] The decision not to treat with PV was originally based on the difficulty of needle placement in these severely collapsed vertebral bodies. However, recent experience suggests that accurate needle introduction into extremely collapsed vertebrae is possible when smaller (13-gauge) needles are used.[13] Furthermore, it was noted that many of the extremely collapsed vertebral bodies are often more collapsed centrally (Fig. 9-4) than laterally. The lateral sparing allows the operating physician to place needles into the remaining lateral trabecular space and to obtain acceptable filling. Patients adequately treated in this manner may experience good pain relief.[13] Even so, treating extremely collapsed vertebral bodies is more challenging than treating vertebral bodies with less height loss, and it likely carries a greater risk of technical or clinical failure. Patients with such conditions should be made aware of these risks, and the operating physician should attempt PV for such extreme cases of collapse only after gaining substantial experience with more routine cases.

References

1. Chiras J, Depriester C, Weill A, et al. [Percutaneous vertebral surgery. Technics and indications.] *J Neuroradiol* 1997; 24(1):45–59.
2. Weill A, Chiras J, Simon JM, et al. Spinal metastases: indications for and results of percutaneous injection of acrylic surgical cement. *Radiology* 1996; 199(1):241–247.
3. Cotten A, Dewatre F, Cortet B, et al. Percutaneous vertebroplasty for osteolytic metastases and myeloma: effects of the percentage of lesion filling and the leakage of methyl methacrylate at clinical follow-up. *Radiology* 1996; 200(2):525–530.
4. Jasper LE, Deramond H, Mathis JM, et al. Material properties of various cements for use with vertebroplasty. *J Mater Sci Mater Med* 2002; 13:1–5.

5. Mathis JM, Eckel TS, Belkoff SM, et al. Percutaneous vertebroplasty: a therapeutic option for pain associated with vertebral compression fracture. *J Back Musculoskel Rehab* 1999; 13(1):11–17.
6. Barr JD, Barr MS, Lemley TJ, et al. Percutaneous vertebroplasty for pain relief and spinal stabilization. *Spine* 2000; 25(8):923–928.
7. Gangi A, Kastler BA, Dietemann JL. Percutaneous vertebroplasty guided by a combination of CT and fluoroscopy. *Am J Neuroradiol* 1994; 15(1):83–86.
8. Barr JD, Barr MS, Lemley TJ. CT as the sole imaging modality for performance of percutaneous vertebroplasty. Poster presented at the 36th Annual Meeting of the American Society of Neuroradiology, Philadelphia, May 17–21, 1998.
9. Barr JD, Barr MS. Coaxial needle system for percutaneous vertebroplasty. Poster presented at the 38th Annual Meeting of the American Society of Neuroradiology, Atlanta, April 3–8, 2000.
10. Kado DM, Browner WS, Palermo L, et al. Vertebral fractures and mortality in older women: a prospective study. Study of Osteoporotic Fractures Research Group. *Arch Intern Med* 1999; 159(11): 1215–1220.
11. Barr JD, Barr MS. Fluoroscopically visible vertebral fracture instability observed during vertebroplasty. Presented at the Joint Annual Meetings of the American Society of Neuroradiology, American Society of Head and Neck Radiology, American Society of Pediatric Neuroradiology, American Society of Interventional and Therapeutic Neuroradiology, and American Society of Spine Radiology, San Diego, May 23–28, 1999.
12. Mathis JM, Petri M, Naff N. Percutaneous vertebroplasty treatment of steroid-induced osteoporotic compression fractures. *Arthritis Rheum* 1998; 41(1):171–175.
13. Barr JD, Mervart M. Percutaneous vertebroplasty of vertebra plana. Poster presented at the 38th Annual Meeting of the American Society of Neuroradiology, Atlanta, April 3–8, 2000.

10

Complications

Hervé Deramond, Jacques E. Dion, and Jacques Chiras

Over the past few years, the percutaneous vertebroplasty (PV) procedure has become increasingly popular throughout the United States and Europe, and its use is now experiencing explosive growth. A plethora of abbreviated technical or "hands-on" courses are now available, and many operating physicians with little or no experience are beginning to treat patients. Indeed, complications that were never seen in the early stages of the development of PV are now being reported; most of these complications are, in fact, preventable. The first essentials are a thorough knowledge of spinal anatomy, image-guided localization, and patient selection criteria. Then, to minimize complications as much as possible, a high-quality fluoroscopy system must be used during the procedure, and the physician must have familiarity with PV tools and cements and adhere to strict sterile technique.

This chapter describes the complications that may be encountered during PV, including incidents, symptoms, imaging findings, and treatment. Use of the knowledge contained in this chapter should enable most physicians to perform PV with a symptomatic complication rate of less than 1% for patients with osteoporosis and vertebral hemangiomas (VHs) and a rate of no more than 5 to 10% for patients with malignant tumors. It should be remembered that *prevention* is key to the safe practice of PV.

Incidents and Complications

Incidents

An incident is an asymptomatic event usually related to a cement leak into paravertebral soft tissues or veins.

Cement Leakage into Paravertebral Soft Tissues

Cement can occasionally flow retrograde along the outside of the cannula and leak into the paravertebral soft tissues (Fig. 10-1). Such leaks are typically asymptomatic and can be prevented in several ways. Using a transpedicular needle approach increases the path length required for the cement to reach the exterior of the vertebral body, thereby decreasing the likelihood of cement leak. When a hammer is used to place needles, there is theoretically closer contact between the needle and the surrounding bone because the needle wobbles less during insertion. Inserting the needle by manually twisting and pushing may widen the introduction path and allow more space between the needle and surrounding bone, thereby facilitating cement leaks. At the end of the procedure, the cement remaining in the cannula can sometimes be inadvertently deposited when the cannula is withdrawn. This extraneous deposit of cement can be avoided by rotating (twisting) the cannula while the cement is polymerizing so that the cement in the cannula is separated from the cement injected into the vertebral body. This maneuver will also prevent the cannula from becoming permanently fixed in the cement bolus inside the vertebral body.

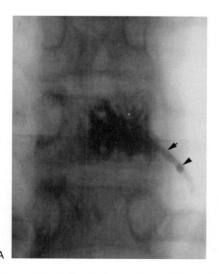 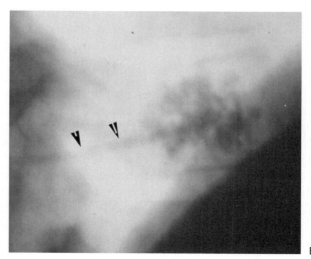

A   B

Figure 10-1. Leak (arrowheads) into the paravertebral soft tissue along the track of the needle after a parapedicular posterolateral approach: (A) AP and (B) lateral views.

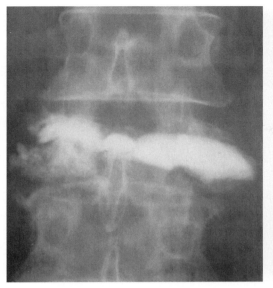 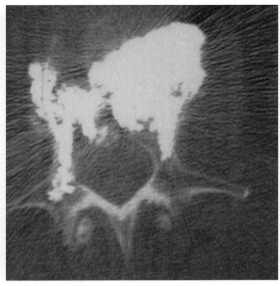

A   B

Figure 10-2. Cement extravasation into the left paravertebral soft tissue through a breach in the vertebral cortex caused by tumor osteolysis. (A) AP view. (B) Axial CT scan.

Cement extravasation into the paravertebral soft tissues can also occur through a breach in the vertebral cortex caused by the initial injury or by tumor osteolysis (Fig. 10-2). Such extravasation, which can be detected and minimized through careful fluoroscopic monitoring in frontal and lateral projections, is rarely problematic.

Cement Leakage into Paravertebral Veins
Cement often leaks into paravertebral veins; however, if the injection is stopped as soon as venous extravasation is fluoroscopically visualized, clinical consequences rarely develop. If the injection is not stopped, there is a risk of pulmonary embolism via the azygous vein or vena cava or of local pain exacerbation.

Cement can also leak into the epidural veins (Fig. 10-3), but, again, such leakage is not associated with clinical problems if the injection is quickly stopped and the leak is small. This type of leak can also be avoided if the operating physician uses good lateral fluoroscopic monitoring and stops the injection as soon as the cement arrives at the projection of the posterior wall. If the cement is allowed to leak into the foraminal veins, it can induce radiculopathy (Fig. 10-4).

The extension of cement into the disk space is not uncommon; it has been observed in up to 20% of PV cases (Fig. 10-5). The cement usually extends through a previously damaged or fractured

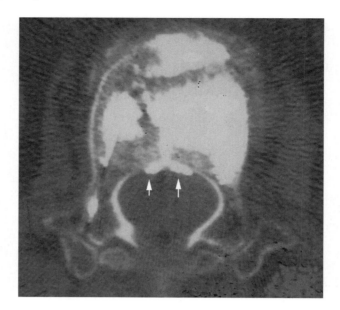

Figure 10-3. Axial CT scan showing cement leak (arrows) into the epidural veins via the basilar vein after PV in a patient with an osteoporotic VCF.

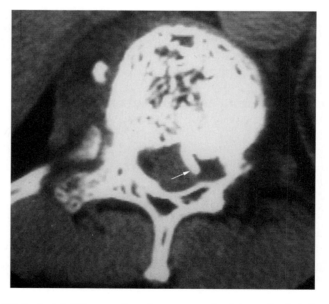

Figure 10-4. Axial CT scan showing cement leak into the left foraminal vein, inducing radiculopathy after PV in a patient with VH.

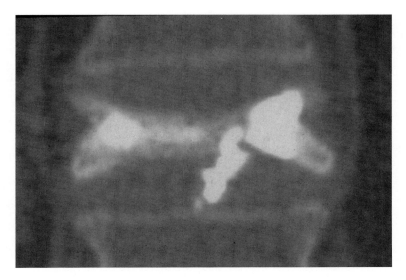

Figure 10-5. Coronal CT scan reconstruction showing cement leak into the disk after PV in a patient with an osteoporotic VCF.

vertebral end plate. Fortunately, most of the patients in whom this leakage occurs remain asymptomatic. Injection of cement into the disk space may contribute to the occurrence of secondary adjacent vertebral collapse in osteoporotic patients. Theoretically, the presence of cement in the disk would be expected to increase the apparent stiffness of the disk and thereby alter the normal spine kinematics at the injected level. The altered kinematic state may place additional stress on the adjacent level, putting those levels at risk for fracture. This point remains unproven at the present time

Complications

Complications, adverse events requiring treatment or prolongation of hospital stay, occur less frequently than incidents. The complication rate is related to the specific indication for PV treatment. When PV is used to treat osteoporotic vertebral compression fractures (VCFs) or VHs, the incidence of symptomatic complications is less than 1% (Table 10-1), whereas complication rates range from 5 to 10% when PV is performed to treat vertebral bodies that are infiltrated with malignant neoplasms (Table 10-2).[1] Complications can be related to the percutaneous approach, the medical condition of the patient, and the injection of polymethylmethacrylate (PMMA).

Spinal Infection

Spinal infection appears to be rare, as only one case of this complication has been reported.[1] That patient treated with PV de-

TABLE 10-1 Complications of Percutaneous Vertebroplasty in Osteoporotic Vertebral Fractures and Vertebral Hemangiomas (VH)

Parameter	Osteoporotic vertebral fractures					VH
	Grados et al.[5]	Jensen et al.[3]	Cortet et al.[6]	Cyteval et al.[7]	Chiras and Deramond[1]	Deramond et al.[8]
Number of patients	25	29	16	20	67	54
Number of PVs	34	47	20	23	76	55
Transitory worsening of the pain	1	0	0	0	1	0
Transitory fever	2	NS[a]	0	0	NS[a]	0
Transitory radiculopathy	2	0	0	0	1	2
Durable radiculopathy	0	0	0	1	1	0
Rib fracture	0	2	0	0	0	0
Infection	0	0	0	0	0	0
Spinal cord compression	0	0	0	0	0	0

[a]Not specified.

veloped an infection (spondylitis) and presented with worsening back pain and fever a few weeks after the procedure. Treatment consisted of 3 months of medical management with intravenous antibiotics and immobilization, after which the infection completely resolved. Of course, the specific treatment plan for spinal infection depends on the imaging findings and the presence or absence of neurological symptoms. Patients at high risk of infection because of poor medical status or who are immunocompromised should be given antibiotics prophylactically. Immunocompromise may be the only indication for antibiotics added to the cement.

TABLE 10-2 Complications of Percutaneous Vertebroplasty for Malignant Tumors in the Spine

Parameter	Investigators		
	Weill et al.[9]	Cotten et al.[10]	Chiras and Deramond[1]
Number of patients	37	37	113
Number of PVs	52	40	120
Transitory worsening of the pain	2	1	2
Transitory fever	NS[a]	0	NS[a]
Transitory radiculopathy	1	1	5
Durable radiculopathy	2	2	5
Infection	0	0	1
Spinal cord compression	0	0	1

[a]Not specified.

Transitory Increase in Pain

Transitory increase in pain is infrequent ($< 2\%$)[2] and may be related to manipulation during the procedure, injection of the cement at high pressure, or inflammatory reactions induced by the presence of the cement. In any case, such pain, in our experience, typically resolves in less than 48 h with the use of nonsteroidal antiinflammatory medications.

Transitory Fever

Transitory fever is rare and may be related to the causes of transitory increase in pain just mentioned. In our experience, the fever resolves in less than 48 h after a course of nonsteroidal antiinflammatory medications.

Rib Fractures

There is only one report of rib fracture after PV in the literature: the two fractures (one each in two osteoporotic patients) were attributed to the manual method of needle insertion.[3] The fractures were likely a result of the thorax being compressed against the procedure table during needle insertion. In osteoporotic patients, it is not unreasonable to expect rib fractures to result from such compression. Theoretically, these fractures may be prevented by tapping the needle with a small hammer to effect insertion. However, it must be noted that the efficacy of this insertion technique at reducing rib fractures has not been tested and that some patients experience more pain with the tapping than with the manual method of insertion.

Radiculopathy

Radiculopathy is related to the leakage of cement into the foraminal veins or the foraminal space.[1] It usually resolves after local injection of steroids and anesthetic or after medical treatment with oral nonsteroidal antiinflammatory medications. In rare instances, however, radiculopathies are recalcitrant to medical treatment and require surgical excision of the foraminal cement. Such radiculopathies are more often associated with malignant tumors (3–5%) than with the other indications ($< 1\%$) because the former is associated with larger leaks.

Spinal Cord Compression

The literature reports one case of spinal cord compression, which occurred in a patient with a spinal metastasis.[1] In fact, the patient had had clinical symptoms of spinal cord compression before the PV procedure, but the neurological signs were accentuated after PV. Emergent surgical excision of the epidural cement was performed, and complete recovery was obtained. However, the number of anecdotal reports of this extreme complication has increased as more PVs are being performed by less experienced operating physicians.

Symptomatic Pulmonary Embolism

One case of symptomatic pulmonary embolism, which occurred immediately after PV, has been described in the literature.[4] This complication can result from excessive cement injection or extravasation into the paravertebral veins. Symptomatic pulmonary embolus requires medical management by a pulmonary specialist with supportive medical therapy and anticoagulation.

Hemorrhage

Hemorrhage can occur in patients with coagulopathy. One of the authors treated a patient with such a complication (H.D., unpublished data). That patient presented with myeloma, hypercalcemia, and severe pain. In spite of coagulation disorders, PV was indicated before chemotherapy to provide pain relief and to allow the patient to remain ambulatory. PV was performed with a single needle, using a parapedicular approach. Three days later, the patient complained of abdominal pain, and a CT scan revealed a retroperitoneal hematoma related to leakage of blood secondary to the needle puncture. The puncture was sealed by injecting glue via a transpedicular percutaneous route (Fig. 10-6).

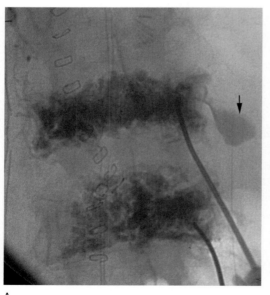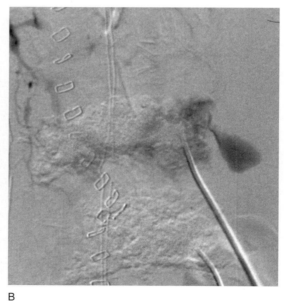

A   B

Figure 10-6. This patient presented with retroperitoneal hematoma 2 days after a PV performed via a parapedicular route at two vertebral levels. Contrast was injected via an 18-gauge needle inserted into the pedicle. (A) Nonsubtracted transosseous venogram showing leak of contrast medium through the previous parapedicular hole (arrow). (B) Subtracted image. The puncture was sealed by injecting glue via the needle.

In general, whenever possible, coagulation disorders should be corrected before PV.

Death

To date, the literature has recorded no report of a death related to PV. However, there is an anecdotal report of two deaths secondary to prophylactic PV for a large number of vertebrae (7 in one patient, 10 in the other) during a single procedure. Although the cause of death has yet to be confirmed, physicians must take into consideration the potential pulmonary compromise resulting from the concurrent treatment of an excessive number of vertebrae. It is recommended that no more than three levels be treated with PV during a single procedure.

References

1. Chiras J, Deramond H. Complications des vertebroplasties. In: Saillant G, Laville C, eds. *Echecs et Complications de la Chirurgie du Rachis. Chirurgie de Reprise.* Paris: Sauramps Medical; 1995:149–153.
2. Chiras J, Depriester C, Weill A, et al. [Percutaneous vertebral surgery. Technics and indications.] *J Neuroradiol* 1997; 24(1):45–59.
3. Jensen ME, Evans AJ, Mathis JM, et al. Percutaneous polymethyl methacrylate vertebroplasty in the treatment of osteoporotic vertebral body compression fractures: technical aspects. *Am J Neuroradiol* 1997; 18(10):1897–1904.
4. Padovani B, Kasriel O, Brunner P, et al. Pulmonary embolism caused by acrylic cement: a rare complication of percutaneous vertebroplasty. *Am J Neuroradiol* 1999; 20(3):375–377.
5. Grados F, Depriester C, Cayrolle G, et al. Long-term observations of vertebral osteoporotic fractures treated by percutaneous vertebroplasty. *Rheumatology* 2000; 39:1410–1414.
6. Cortet B, Cotten A, Boutry N, et al. Percutaneous vertebroplasty in the treatment of osteoporotic vertebral compression fractures: an open prospective study. *J Rheumatol* 1999; 26(10):2222–2228.
7. Cyteval C, Sarrabere MP, Roux JO, et al. Acute osteoporotic vertebral collapse: open study on percutaneous injection of acrylic surgical cement in 20 patients. *Am J Roentgenol* 1999; 173(6):1685–1690.
8. Deramond H, Depriester C, Galibert P, et al. Percutaneous vertebroplasty with polymethyl methacrylate. Technique, indications, and results. *Radiol Clin North Am* 1998; 36(3):533–546.
9. Weill A, Chiras J, Simon JM, et al. Spinal metastases: indications for and results of percutaneous injection of acrylic surgical cement. *Radiology* 1996; 199(1):241–247.
10. Cotten A, Dewatre F, Cortet B, et al. Percutaneous vertebroplasty for osteolytic metastases and myeloma: effects of the percentage of lesion filling and the leakage of methyl methacrylate at clinical follow-up. *Radiology* 1996; 200(2):525–530.

11

Starting a Clinical Practice

Wayne J. Olan and John M. Mathis

Developing a successful clinical practice in percutaneous verte-broplasty (PV) can be a challenging and multifaceted task. Requirements include physician training and education, institutional preparation, marketing of the practice, selecting an appropriate first patient, and support systems for patient tracking and quality assurance.

Physician Training and Education

Because PV is a relatively new procedure, most physicians will not have received training in this procedure during their residency and fellowship. Therefore, most practitioners will need to obtain training through some form of continuing medical education. Training recommendations are described by the American College of Radiology in the Standard for the Performance of Percutaneous Vertebroplasty (Appendix I). According to those standards, the well-trained resident or fellow should have (1) successfully performed no fewer than five supervised procedures, (2) attended lectures that provided important details about pertinent anatomy, selection and use of image guidance, patient selection and preparation, complications and contraindications of PV, materials needed for the procedure, and the appropriate handling and preparation of biomaterials, and (3) reviewed the literature pertaining to PV, including PV-related biomaterials and biomechanical data.

Physicians in practice may obtain training by attending a dedicated one-day course that includes didactic instruction covering the various aspects of the procedure, similar to that just mentioned for residents and fellows, and hands-on cadaver training for image guidance, needle placement, and cement preparation. After completing this training, the physician should successfully perform at least two PV procedures proctored by a trained physician. Adherence to these requirements will set a reasonable minimum standard for physicians wishing to begin performing PV.

In addition, the physician wishing to perform PV should be knowledgeable about osteoporosis because it is the most common cause of vertebral compression fractures (VCFs) in patients who will be treated with PV. Physicians performing the procedure should be able to educate patients about the disease process and ways to prevent subsequent VCFs. If the physician's practice does not include experience with all aspects of the medical management of osteoporosis, from diagnosis to pharmacological treatment, it may be wise to establish a team approach to address the needs of patients with this disease process. Percutaneous vertebroplasy treats the pain of the VCF, but it does not address osteoporosis. Osteoporosis is a systemic disease and the patient with osteoporosis needs ongoing evaluation and care to minimize the risk of future fracture and debilitation.

Institutional Preparation

Adequate preparation by the sponsoring institution is important to ensure a successful PV program. First, the institution is responsible for the credentialing of all physicians who will perform PV. Therefore, criteria for certification, based on the American College of Radiology's Standard for the Performance of Percutaneous Vertebroplasty (Appendix I) must be established, and the completion of such training must be documented. Second, the institution must have adequate equipment and personnel resources. Performing PV requires high-quality image guidance equipment (see Chapter 6 for details). Support personnel needs to be provided with training consistent with their roles during the PV procedures. Radiographic technologists must be familiar with imaging equipment and must obtain and stock all materials necessary for the procedure. Nursing personnel must provide monitoring, supportive care, and conscious sedation during the procedure, as well as postprocedure monitoring for restricted activity and possible complications; they must also instruct the patient and family about care of the operative site, medication regimens, and what to do in the event of problems.

It is a good idea to build automatic follow-up into the routine of patient care. This goal can be accomplished by a simple telephone call 24 h after the procedure, which can be repeated if the patient did not report good pain relief at the first follow-up call. This information should be maintained for all patients and should provide the basis for quality assessment and improvement.

Members of the PV team will be faced with scheduling, billing, patient and family questions, and data collection (history and physical as well as previous radiographic images). All members of the PV team need to be informed about the basics of the procedure (what it is called, the indications for PV, information needed for patient evaluation, etc.). Attention to such details at the initial practice setup will increase patient and referring physician satisfaction.

Marketing the Procedure and the Practice

Physician awareness of the advantages and availability of any new procedure is essential to a successful start-up. One must find an effective method of identifying, contacting, and establishing a referral base. Referral sources for PV include (but are not limited to) the specialties of family practice, rheumatology, rehabilitation medicine, pain anesthesia, orthopedics, neurosurgery, oncology, transplant surgery, and geriatrics. Any of these physicians may need help in the management of patients with painful VCFs. Getting the message to these physicians may be accomplished through personal contact, continuing medical education seminars, medical staff meetings, brochures, local newsletters, and Internet web pages (e.g., spinefracture.com). Because each of these methods may reach a different group, it is recommended that any and all available methods be used, including the simple expedient of referring interested physicians and patients to scientific articles about PV.

Concentration of effort should not be limited to the medical community but should extend to the general public as well. Because many physicians (and patients) may be skeptical about the benefits of PV if they have no personal experience with the pain relief it can afford, it is important to put additional effort into providing local radio, television, and newspaper services with accounts of successful procedures and with names and telephone numbers members of the public can use to access additional information. Other avenues include lectures at church gatherings, presentations at health symposia, and informal talks to senior citizen groups.

These marketing methods often produce a large volume of telephone calls and questions about the procedure and whether particular situations are appropriate for its use (i.e., chronic VCFs, back pain, and degenerative disk disease). Especially at first, answering such questions will take a lot of time and energy on the part of the practice's team. To respond to such requests, there should be at least one designated person who understands the criteria for patient selection and what information is needed for evaluating patients who seem appropriate. A website or pamphlets that explain the procedure, selection criteria, and risk and benefits will streamline the referral program and save a tremendous amount of time.

Selecting the First Patient

When performed by experienced physicians, PV is generally a simple procedure with few complications.[1–6] However, the beginning practitioner must be aware of the complexities of the start-up situation. First, as with all medical procedures, there is a definite learning curve and the risk of complications will be higher for the new practitioner. Second, some referred patients will have had numerous chronic VCFs and may be generally in poor health; such a patient is not the best candidate for a new PV practice.

Initially, the practitioner should avoid patients with radicular components to the pain history, substantial back pain before the VCFs (which may be related to degenerative disk disease or spinal stenosis), pain not easily localized to the fracture to be treated, or history and physical examinations that do not correlate with the compression injuries. In addition, it is a good idea to reserve treating patients with metastatic VCFs until experience with osteoporotic fractures has been gained. The incidence of cement leak is 5 to 10 times higher in patients with metastatic disease than in those with osteoporosis.[7] The former also tend to have less pain relief with PV. Although selected patients with metastatic fractures are appropriate candidates for PV, such patients should not form part of the basis of a new practice. Finally, the new practitioner should focus on patients with single-level rather than multiple-level fractures. Patients selected for PV with multiple VCFs should be treated only at symptomatic levels that can be correlated to definite acute finding by magnetic resonance (MR) imaging or nuclear medicine. It should be remembered there is currently no indication to treat prophylactically.

Thus, ideally, the first patient should be one who had been ambulatory and doing well before experiencing the fracture. The fracture should be relatively acute (2–6 weeks old), and the patient should have continued pain that limits normal activities of daily living or requires substantial analgesic therapy. The physical examination should show a good correlation between the pain location and the VCF to be treated. If the patient has had VCFs before, MR imaging should be used as part of the initial workup to confirm which fracture is truly acute, and only that level should be treated with PV. With such a patient, the probability of providing substantial pain relief with PV is high.

Support Systems for Patient Tracking and Quality Improvement

All patients should be in the care of an appropriate primary physician who will ensure long-term follow-up and therapy for underlying medical conditions such as osteoporosis or neoplasm. Such physicians may make up the original referral base. However, the self-referred patient (see Chapter 4) needs to be directed into a network that ensures quality ongoing care.

In the established practice that efficiently manages clinical situations, implementing PV as a new procedure will be relatively easy. However, for the practice without a definite clinical component, the addition of PV will be a big change. It may ultimately be helpful to have a PV clinic that is dedicated to seeing new patients and providing follow-up for those already treated. The physician must be prepared to establish a pathway for questions and inquiries; to avoid patient frustration and anger, there should be a dedicated individual in the institution who is easily accessible.

Patient scheduling may be divided into three categories: pre-procedure consultations, procedure scheduling, and follow-up visits. Staff members should be able to direct patients into one of the categories and exclude patients who have unrelated problems. It is also helpful to develop clinical practice guidelines for PV and establish before-, during-, and after-procedure care protocols for the patient. For example, a preprocedure checklist can be a valuable tool. The preprocedure consultation provides the physician and staff members the opportunity to explain the PV procedure to the patient and his or her family. Patients are instructed to bring all their pertinent medical records and recent imaging studies for the consultation. At the time of this consultation, all necessary laboratory tests (such as coagulation studies) may be ordered. If additional imaging studies (such as MR imaging or nuclear medicine) are needed, then they can be scheduled at that time as well. A carefully selected and well-prepared patient will increase the potential for a good outcome and a satisfied patient.

The follow-up interview may be in person or may be conducted by telephone, usually at 24 h and then at 7 to 14 days after the procedure. The staff person conducting the follow-up interview should obtain and record standardized information for the database and be prepared to answer common questions, which are often related to local treatment site bruising and soreness.

Summary/Conclusions

Obtaining proper training is the first step in developing a successful PV clinical practice. Although organizing institutional support to provide the infrastructure needed to establish a PV practice, and then marketing the practice, may seen like daunting challenges at first, the rewards are great. Careful preparation for and selection of the first patient should aid greatly in a smooth start. After the procedure, timely and accurate patient follow-up will increase the likelihood of patient satisfaction and provide a means of assuring quality patient care. Attention to these details during start-up will prevent patient frustration, will increase referrals, and will make PV a professionally rewarding addition to clinical practice.

References

1. Chiras J, Deramond H. Complications des vertebroplasties. In: Saillant G, Laville C, eds. *Echecs et Complications de la Chirurgie du Rachis. Chirurgie de Reprise*, Paris: Sauramps Medical; 1995:149–153.
2. Cortet B, Cotten A, Boutry N, et al. Percutaneous vertebroplasty in the treatment of osteoporotic vertebral compression fractures: an open prospective study. *J Rheumatol* 1999; 26(10):2222–2228.
3. Cyteval C, Sarrabere MP, Roux JO, et al. Acute osteoporotic vertebral collapse: open study on percutaneous injection of acrylic surgical cement in 20 patients. *Am J Roentgenol* 1999; 173(6):1685–1690.
4. Deramond H, Depriester C, Galibert P, et al. Percutaneous vertebroplasty with polymethyl methacrylate. Technique, indications, and results. *Radiol Clin North Am* 1998; 36(3):533–546.
5. Grados F, Depriester C, Cayrolle G, et al. Long-term observations of vertebral osteoporotic fractures treated by percutaneous vertebroplasty. *Rheumatology* 2000; 39:1410–1414.
6. Jensen ME, Evans AJ, Mathis JM, et al. Percutaneous polymethyl methacrylate vertebroplasty in the treatment of osteoporotic vertebral body compression fractures: technical aspects. *Am J Neuroradiol* 1997; 18(10):1897–1904.
7. Cotten A, Dewatre F, Cortet B, et al. Percutaneous vertebroplasty for osteolytic metastases and myeloma: effects of the percentage of lesion filling and the leakage of methyl methacrylate at clinical follow-up. *Radiology* 1996; 200(2):525–530.

12

Future Directions: Challenges and Research Opportunities

John M. Mathis, Stephen M. Belkoff, and Hervé Deramond

Percutaneous vertebroplasty (PV) has created a tremendous amount of interest among patients, their families, and physicians as a means of addressing problems caused by osteoporosis or neoplasm-induced vertebral compression fractures (VCFs). However, interest in the procedure is not limited to these treatment groups. The introduction of PV in 1984, and its growing acceptance as the standard of care for the treatment of painful VCFs, have encouraged scientific investigations into the palliative mechanisms of the procedure.[1–9] Manufacturers have also been eager to develop new devices to meet the demands of the procedure. In the next decade, we can expect to see a growing body of research that will expand the current knowledge about minimally invasive procedures, including (but not limited to) mechanical augmentation of the spine.[10–13] We anticipate that commercial efforts will follow rapidly, with the development of new devices and materials that enhance and improve our capabilities for these interventions. This chapter presents an overview of what we believe needs to be addressed and where we are likely to see advancements.

New Devices

Since the introduction of PV,[14] there has been a growing interest in developing new devices for the percutaneous delivery of bone cement.[15] Initial design efforts have revolved around addressing the deficiencies of available systems. For instance, the Jamshidi bone biopsy needle has been the preferred system for PV in the United States[16] despite features that made it difficult to use. Such features include a fixed handle that obscures visualization of the needle tip under fluoroscopy, a tapered cannula that limits the amount of cement that can be discharged when the trocar is inserted, and a bevel-point tip geometry that is not advantageous for penetrating cortical bone.

Many manufacturers have now released needles with modified handle designs and locking trocars. A locking trocar ensures that the trocar tip and cannula tip geometry match, and it holds the tip of the needle in place during insertion. Cannulae that are not tapered are preferred for PV because this design eliminates dead space between the trocar and cannula wall, thus enabling the trocar to discharge all the cement upon insertion into the cannula. The ability to inject the remaining cement in the cannula is an important option to have, particularly when the cement becomes very viscous and is no longer easy to inject through the cannula by means of a syringe. Because the trocar diameter is small relative to the plunger of a typical 1-mL syringe, it has a mechanical advantage compared with the syringe, facilitating the delivery of even viscous cement. Depending on the length and diameter of the cannula, as much as 1.0 mL of usable cement may be left in the cannula, which can be delivered by inserting the trocar. Finally, new trocar tip geometries allow easier entry into the bone, regardless of the site selected for access. The original bevel design was prone to slide off the bone if the entry site was at an incline to the tip. Several new tip designs are much more effective at engaging the periosteum and penetrating the vertebral cortex. Additional refinements in needle designs are anticipated, but they are likely to be modest because most of the major design problems have been solved and the designs available work well.

Controlled deposition of cement inside the vertebra during PV is an area with considerable room for improvement. Polymethylmethacrylate (PMMA) is the only material currently used in clinical practice for PV. Although PMMA has been used successfully for many years for PV, its use presents some challenges. Once its components are mixed, PMMA cement has a limited useful working time of 5 to 10 min. During that time, as the cement begins to polymerize, its viscosity and handling characteristics change, and the cement becomes progressively more difficult to inject. This difficulty may be partially overcome by adding more monomer to the cement mixture, thereby decreasing its viscosity and increasing its working time.[16,17] Alternatively, the cement may be injected under higher pressure, such as is developed with small syringes (1 mL) or injection devices. The injection devices currently available are expensive and have the disadvantage of providing less control over injection than is possible with the syringe. With any of the injection devices, once cement begins to flow (typically through a long tube connecting the device to the percutaneously placed needle), there is no mechanism for rapidly releasing pressure in the system and immediately stopping cement flow. Therefore, there can be a delay between detecting extravasation and the cessation of cement injection. An optimal injection device should offer enough mechanical advantage to permit easy cement injection of controllable amounts (e.g., 0.1–0.2 mL at a time) and to prevent clinically significant extravasation. Injection of small incremental volumes not only helps prevent extravasation, but also prevents the pain often experienced by conscious patients when larger volumes are injected rapidly.

Currently, the deposition location of cement is only partially controllable. Even though the needle is carefully placed and constant fluoroscopic monitoring is used during injection, the cement (which flows along the path of least resistance) can still extravasate outside the vertebra or into a blood vessel.[16,18] However, when extravasation is noted, it can be stopped by halting injection. Devices that would enable the clinician to deposit cement precisely and to customize the distribution of cement within the vertebral body would be a substantial improvement over existing systems.

Currently, clinicians empirically select the volume of cement to be injected into a VCF. A recent study reports the volume of cement needed to restore strength and stiffness to various vertebral levels.[8] Cement volume alone, however, was not well correlated to mechanical property restoration. Restoration of mechanical properties also likely depends on bone density. Thus, a more sophisticated algorithm needs to be developed to predict the volume of cement needed to restore strength and stiffness based on the material properties of the cement chosen for injection and on the geometry and material properties of the vertebral body to be injected.

The inflatable bone tamp has created considerable interest in height restoration after VCF (see Chapter 7). Other methods of height restoration are likely to follow. Ex vivo biomechanical evaluation of the tamp device indicates that significant height can be restored,[6,7] but it is unknown if such restorations can be obtained clinically. Preliminary clinical results suggest that only modest height restoration has been attained with the bone tamp, perhaps in part because one patient selection criterion includes patients with weeks-old fractures. A VCF in the process of healing probably resists tamp inflation and inhibits height restoration. The outcomes of other methods or devices that apply spinal traction to obtain partial or complete vertebral height restoration before cementing will likely also be affected by the time delay between fracture and treatment.

New Cements and Biomaterials

As stated earlier, the only cements now in use for PV are various types of PMMA. None of these are approved by the Food and Drug Administration (FDA) for the specific purpose of PV, and none contains an opacifier in sufficient quantity to make the cement easily seen on fluoroscopy during percutaneous injection.[9] Used successfully for decades in orthopedic practice, PMMAs therefore represent a relatively old cement technology. Their material properties are greater in compression than in tension or shear,[19] which seems appropriate for use in mechanically augmenting vertebral bodies. Another positive attribute of the PMMA-type cements is the rapid setting time, which allows the possibility of weight bearing within a matter of hours after cement injection. Approximately 90% of the strength of PMMA cement is attained within an hour of mixing.[19]

Despite these positive attributes, there are several PMMA properties that need improvement. Polymethylmethacrylate cements are not intrinsically opaque.[9] Concerns remain about the potential for local thermal necrosis created by the exothermic heat generated during polymerization and about cytotoxicity from the free monomer left unbound during the polymerization process.[4,20,21] Furthermore, PMMA cements are not bioactive and, therefore, do not promote bone ingrowth or remodeling over time. Once polymerized, PMMA is difficult to drill and tap for screw placement, should subsequent orthopedic hardware be required for the spine.

Ideally, the development of new cements should address the deficiencies of existing PMMA cements. For instance, calcium phosphate cements are resorbable. The composition of this class of cements is very similar to the mineral component of bone and, as such, it may serve as a building block for local bone regeneration and remodeling through osteoblastic activity. Whether this regeneration could occur when the process of bone production and repair is altered pathologically (i.e., osteoporosis) has yet to be evaluated. Adding bone stimulants, such as bone morphogenic proteins, to the resorbable cement could potentially aid the remodeling process. Hydroxyapatite cement has the added advantage of no exothermic reaction and no monomer release. Additionally, hydroxyapatite cements are intrinsically radiopaque, so they need no additional opacification (Fig. 12-1). Disadvantages of hydroxyapatite cements include lower tensile and shear strengths and longer cure times compared with PMMA. Maximum compressive strength, for example, is typically achieved over a 24-h period. The theoretical advantages of a resorbable cement will have to be weighed against the cost of an increased non–weight-bearing postinjection period.

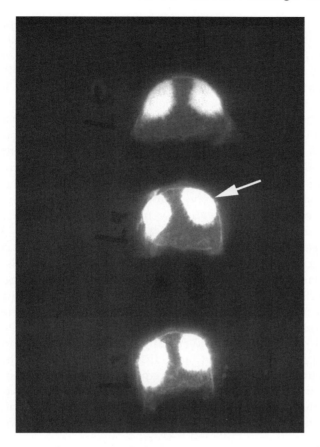

Figure 12-1. Hydroxyapatite-forming cements are now injectable and show promise for use with PV. This class of cements is also naturally radiopaque (example indicated by arrow).

Mechanical demands on vertebrae are primarily compressive, and hydroxyapatite cements are well suited to resist these forces. Although there is concern about the adequacy of various cements and cement volumes to augment vertebrae mechanically, to our knowledge there are no reports elucidating the magnitude of augmentation needed clinically. Therefore, these agents may offer adequate augmentation to treat painful VCFs successfully. Until a controlled, prospective study is conducted to determine what is required for sufficient mechanical augmentation, the question of mechanical sufficiency will remain unanswered.

The use of resorbable cements also begs the question of the value of prophylactic augmentation. If this class of cements fully resorbs or remodels into bone, it may offer a means of mechanical augmentation without the negative aspect of implanting a permanent foreign body into the spine. However, prophylactic augmentation requires the identification of vertebral bodies at risk for fracture. Current methods for predicting vertebral body fracture using dual-energy x-ray absorptiometry (DEXA) or quantitative computed tomography (QCT) are not accurate enough to be effective or financially justified.[22,23]

Another cement property that may be desirable is osseointegration. Rather than resorbing or remodeling, there may be a place in PV for cements, such as bioactive glass cements,[2,24] to chemically or mechanically bond with bone. Bone ingrowth or attachment to the cement would be expected to improve the interface strength between bone and the cement. This potential attribute may be of less value for treatment of VCFs because the cement is in a contained space, and loosening (as may be seen with instrument implantation) is not an issue. Ingrowth could be potentially beneficial in other bone areas when cement is used to anchor materials and fasteners in osteoporotic or damaged bone.

New PMMA cements that have extended working times and have a more appropriate level of opacification compared with the currently available cements would be beneficial. One of us (J.M.M.) has doubled the usual room temperature work time of Simplex P (Stryker-Howmedica-Osteonics, Rutherford, NJ), mixed in accordance with the manufacturer's recommendations, by chilling the cement once it is mixed. Opacification has typically been achieved with barium sulfate. Approximately 30% of barium sulfate by weight is needed in PV for easy and safe monitoring with fluoroscopy.[9] Other opacification agents, such as powdered tungsten and tantalum[25] or zirconium dioxide,[9] may be used as well. The amount of these agents needed for use in PV has not yet been determined in clinical or laboratory investigations.

Robotic Guidance

To date, PV has been performed completely as a manual process. In the future, computer guidance and image analysis may contribute to improving the existing process. These advances could include computer analysis of the vertebra (after fracture) that could give an estimate of the residual internal volume to be filled with cement. Currently, fill volumes are determined empirically by the practitioner, and the amounts selected are completely subjective. They are not based on biomechanical requirements for restoring strength or stiffness of the vertebral body. Analytical analysis could improve the practitioner's ability to choose the minimum volume of cement needed to reinforce a vertebra biomechanically and reduce the overfilling that increases the risk of cement leaks.

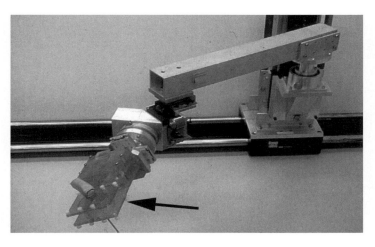

Figure 12-2. Prototype of a robotic arm intended for needle guidance in PV. It was made with a radiolucent needle holder (arrow) for fluoroscopic monitoring of the needle trajectory.

Computer guidance and robotics are making inroads into clinical medicine, including in the operating room. This technology could be used in PV to predict the best trajectory for needle placement and, ultimately, to help guide the needle. A prototype of a robotic delivery system (Fig. 12-2)[26] has analyzed the radiographic appearance of the vertebra in at least two projections and calculated a safe needle trajectory. A robotic arm incorporated a rigid radiolucent needle holder, allowing targeting under fluoroscopic guidance, and constrained the needle to the chosen trajectory during introduction. This simple project was intended as a proof-of-concept experiment to demonstrate what potentially could be achieved with a more refined mechanism. Full automation of the robotic arm and needle introduction are obvious extensions of this research effort.

Alternate Sites for Bone Augmentation

To date, vertebral bodies have been the focus of most of the interest as the site of percutaneous augmentation using bone cement. However, they are not the only site for potential percutaneous treatment. Reports have described good pain relief from percutaneous cement injections in patients suffering from neoplastic invasion and destruction of the pelvis.[27,28] These patients received percutaneous augmentation in areas destroyed by tumor invasion, typically in the supraacetabular region, where weakening caused pain with weight bearing. A similar augmentation (Fig. 12-3) has been performed by one of us (J.M.M.). The

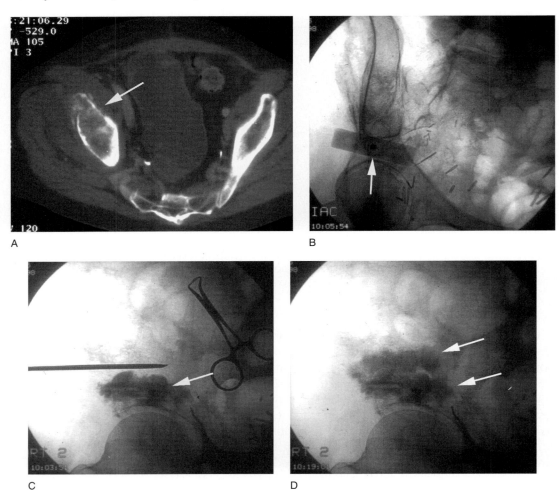

Figure 12-3. This patient experienced pelvic pain with weight bearing. (A) CT scan of the pelvis showing neoplastic destruction of the right supraacetabular region (arrow). (B) Oblique view (looking down the needle—arrow) used for guidance during needle introduction and before cement injection. (C) AP view showing radiopaque cement that has been deposited in the supraacetabular area (arrow). The needle has been moved to a second site for additional cement injection. (D) Final image showing cement in the supraacetabular region after two separate injections (arrows). The patient experienced good pain relief and was able to bear weight on the right hip after this therapy.

patient, who was unable to bear weight before this therapy, reported good pain relief postoperatively that allowed partial weight bearing. An additional opportunity in the pelvic region is treatment of sacral insufficiency fractures. Such treatment of fractures of these types has not been exhaustively investigated and needs further clinical study. Among the questions that still need answering are those involving the best route of cement administration, the type of image guidance needed, the amount of cement required to effect pain relief, and the potential for complications. This prospect is an exciting area of potential therapy because sacral insufficiency fractures, like vertebral fractures before PV, currently have no therapy except management by pain medication and bed rest. The patient may be incapacitated during a long period of convalescence (several weeks to months).

Prophylactic Therapy

Prophylactic therapy of vertebrae that are intact but believed to be at risk of fracture is not currently indicated. Several hurdles need to be overcome before this therapy can be conducted safely. Primary among these obstacles is the need for a method to predict accurately which vertebrae are most likely to fracture.

Another area that may benefit from minimally invasive, prophylactic augmentation is the osteoporotic femoral neck.[29] As with VCFs, the likelihood of hip fracture cannot be predicted accurately. Once a hip fracture has occurred, however, the risk of a similar fracture on the contralateral hip increases dramatically[30] and may be the indication for prophylactic augmentation. Clearly, fundamental research needs to be conducted to determine the efficacy of such a theoretical treatment.

Preoperative Augmentations

It is well reported that instrumentation placed into an osteoporotic spine may fail secondary to low bone density and poor purchase of the orthopedic hardware.[31-33] In addition, because of the rigidity of the instrumented vertebral levels relative to adjacent levels, vertebrae above the levels instrumented are at risk for fracture.[34] Preoperative prophylactic augmentation (Fig. 12-4) of the levels at risk of fracture due to the altered kinematics caused by the instrumentation may be indicated. This procedure can be performed before surgery on an outpatient basis and theoretically should decrease the fracture rate in adjacent vertebrae, but a prospective clinical series is needed to establish its efficacy. Furthermore, the bony purchase of pedicle screws and other hardware can be increased by introducing cement into the area of desired screw placement before screw insertion (Fig. 12-5).[35] For this procedure, PMMA cement is not an optimal material because the cement, once polymerized, becomes brittle and often fractures when hardware is inserted (Fig. 12-4A). Furthermore, PMMA is not easily machined, so drilling and tapping procedures are difficult. However, PMMA can provide satisfactory augmented screw purchase if the screw is inserted into the cement before it polymerizes.

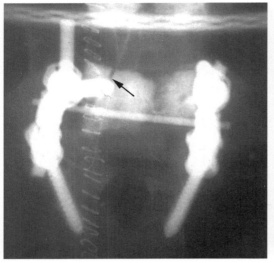
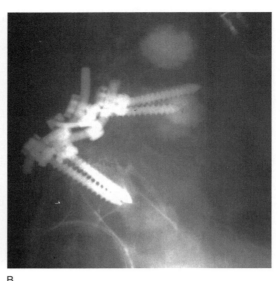

A   B

Figure 12-4. (A) AP and (B) lateral views showing pedicle screw internal fixation at L4-S1 in a patient known to have severe osteoporosis. Preoperative PV was performed at L3 and L4. The L3 level was augmented in an attempt to avoid future VCF. L4 was injected to give better purchase for the pedicle screw in osteoporotic bone. Note the fracture (A, arrow) in the cement at L4 created by the pedicle screw.

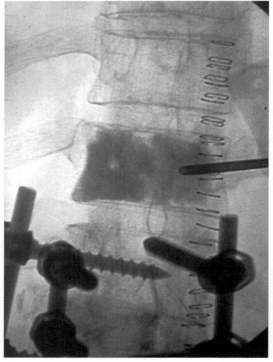
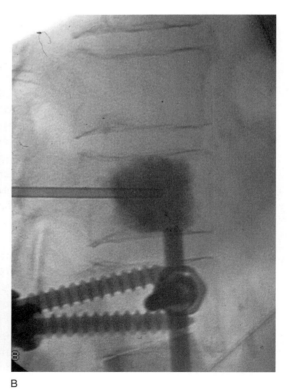

A   B

Figure 12-5. (A) AP and (B) lateral views showing a PV procedure performed with cement above orthopedic hardware in a patient with known osteoporosis. This was done in an attempt to minimize the risk of VCF above the instrumentation.

Summary/Conclusions

Percutaneous vertebroplasty is rapidly becoming the standard of care for the pain associated with VCFs. However, its current application in the spine may be just the beginning of an evolutionary change in the way some bone diseases are treated (i.e., with minimally invasive therapy). New methods for guidance will become available, as will new tools and biomaterials that improve and advance this procedure. The future holds great promise for research and innovation to lead us into new realms of patient care and disease management.

References

1. Tohmeh AG, Mathis JM, Fenton DC, et al. Biomechanical efficacy of unipedicular versus bipedicular vertebroplasty for the management of osteoporotic compression fractures. *Spine* 1999; 24(17):1772–1776.
2. Belkoff SM, Mathis JM, Erbe EM, et al. Biomechanical evaluation of a new bone cement for use in vertebroplasty. *Spine* 2000; 25(9): 1061–1064.
3. Belkoff SM, Maroney M, Fenton DC, et al. An in vitro biomechanical evaluation of bone cements used in percutaneous vertebroplasty. *Bone* 1999; 25(2 suppl):23S–26S.
4. Deramond H, Wright NT, Belkoff SM. Temperature elevation caused by bone cement polymerization during vertebroplasty. *Bone* 1999; 25(2 suppl):17S–21S.
5. Jasper LE, Deramond H, Mathis JM, et al. The effect of monomer-to-powder ratio on the material properties of Cranioplastic. *Bone* 1999; 25(2 suppl):27S–29S.
6. Wilson DR, Myers ER, Mathis JM, et al. Effect of augmentation on the mechanics of vertebral wedge fractures. *Spine* 2000; 25(2):158–165.
7. Belkoff SM, Mathis JM, Fenton DC, et al. An ex vivo biomechanical evaluation of an inflatable bone tamp used in the treatment of compression fracture. *Spine* 2001; 26(2):151–156.
8. Belkoff SM, Mathis JM, Jasper LE, et al. The biomechanics of vertebroplasty: the effect of cement volume on mechanical behavior. *Spine* 2001; 26(14):1537–1541.
9. Jasper LE, Deramond H, Mathis JM, et al. Material properties of various cements for use with vertebroplasty. *J Mater Sci Mater Med* 2002; 13:1–5.
10. Bostrom MP, Lane JM. Future directions. Augmentation of osteoporotic vertebral bodies. *Spine* 1997; 22(24 suppl):38S–42S.
11. Schildhauer TA, Bennett AP, Wright TM, et al. Intravertebral body reconstruction with an injectable in situ–setting carbonated apatite: biomechanical evaluation of a minimally invasive technique. *J Orthop Res* 1999; 17(1):67–72.
12. Bai B, Jazrawi LM, Kummer FJ, et al. The use of an injectable, biodegradable calcium phosphate bone substitute for the prophylactic augmentation of osteoporotic vertebrae and the management of vertebral compression fractures. *Spine* 1999; 24(15):1521–1526.

13. Wehrli FW, Ford JC, Haddad JG. Osteoporosis: clinical assessment with quantitative MR imaging in diagnosis. *Radiology* 1995; 196(3): 631–641.

14. Galibert P, Deramond H, Rosat P, et al. [Preliminary note on the treatment of vertebral angioma by percutaneous acrylic vertebroplasty.] *Neurochirurgie* 1987; 33(2):166–168.

15. Al-Assir I, Perez-Higueras A, Florensa J, et al. Percutaneous vertebroplasty: a special syringe for cement injection. *Am J Neuroradiol* 2000; 21(1):159–161.

16. Jensen ME, Evans AJ, Mathis JM, et al. Percutaneous polymethylmethacrylate vertebroplasty in the treatment of osteoporotic vertebral body compression fractures: technical aspects. *Am J Neuroradiol* 1997; 18(10):1897–1904.

17. Deramond H, Depriester C, Galibert P, et al. Percutaneous vertebroplasty with polymethyl methacrylate. Technique, indications, and results. *Radiol Clin North Am* 1998; 36(3):533–546.

18. Padovani B, Kasriel O, Brunner P, et al. Pulmonary embolism caused by acrylic cement: a rare complication of percutaneous vertebroplasty. *Am J Neuroradiol* 1999; 20(3):375–377.

19. Saha S, Pal S. Mechanical properties of bone cement: a review. *J Biomed Mater Res* 1984; 18(4):435–462.

20. Wenda K, Scheuermann H, Weitzel E, et al. Pharmacokinetics of methyl methacrylate monomer during total hip replacement in man. *Arch Orthop Trauma Surg* 1988; 107(5):316–321.

21. Belkoff SM, Deramond H. The effect of monomer on MCF-7 breast cancer cell viability. Poster presented at the 11th Interdisciplinary Research Conference on Biomaterials (Groupe de Recherches Interdisciplinaire sur les Biomateriaux Ostéo-articulaires Injectables, GRIBOI), March 8–9, 2001.

22. McBroom RJ, Hayes WC, Edwards WT, et al. Prediction of vertebral body compressive fracture using quantitative computed tomography. *J Bone Joint Surg* 1985; 67A:1206–1214.

23. Hayes WC, Piazza SJ, Zysset PK. Biomechanics of fracture risk prediction of the hip and spine by quantitative computed tomography. *Radiol Clin North Am* 1991; 29(1):1–18.

24. Dallap BL, Gadaleta S, Erbe E, et al. Histological, radiological, and mechanical comparison of polymethyl methacrylate (PMMA) and a bioactive bone cement in an ovine model [abstract]. *Trans Orthop Res Soc* 1999; 24:503.

25. Cotten A, Boutry N, Cortet B, et al. Percutaneous vertebroplasty: state of the art. *Radiographics* 1998; 18(2):311–323.

26. Lazarus JA. A computer integrated surgical system for fluoroscopy-guided percutaneous vertebroplasty [thesis]. Johns Hopkins University, Baltimore, MD, 2000.

27. Cotten A, Deprez X, Migaud H, et al. Malignant acetabular osteolyses: percutaneous injection of acrylic bone cement. *Radiology* 1995; 197(1):307–310.

28. Gangi A, Dietemann JL, Schultz A, et al. Interventional radiologic procedures with CT guidance in cancer pain management. *Radiographics* 1996; 16(6):1289–1304.

29. Roubertou H. Étude biomecanique in vitro d'extrémites supérieures

du fémur sans et avec injection intra-osseuse de ciment acrylique. Thesis. Université de Picardie, September 12, 1997.

30. Finsen V, Benum P. Past fractures indicate increased risk of hip fracture. *Acta Orthop Scand* 1986; 57:337–339.

31. Asnis SE, Ernberg JJ, Bostrom MP, et al. Cancellous bone screw thread design and holding power. *J Orthop Trauma* 1996; 10(7):462–469.

32. Chapman JR, Harrington RM, Lee KM, et al. Factors affecting the pullout strength of cancellous bone screws. *J Biomech Eng* 1996; 118(3):391–398.

33. Ruland CM, McAfee PC, Warden KE, et al. Triangulation of pedicular instrumentation. A biomechanical analysis. *Spine* 1991; 16(6 suppl): S270–S276.

34. Kostuik JP, Heggeness MH. Surgery of the osteoporotic spine. In: Frymoyer JW, ed. *The Adult Spine: Principles and Practice.* 2nd ed. Philadelphia: Lippincott-Raven; 1997:1639–1664.

35. Heller KD, Zilkens KW, Hammer J, et al. Does the anchorage form and depth influence the pull-out strength of screws from bone cement? An experimental study. *Arch Orthop Trauma Surg* 1997; 116(1–2):88–91.

List of Abbreviations

ABR	American Board of Radiology
ACGME	Accreditation Council for Graduate Medical Education
ACR	American College of Radiology
ALARA	as low as reasonably achievable
AP	anteroposterior
ARRT	American Registry of Radiologic Technologists
ASTM	American Society for Testing and Materials
BMD	bone mineral density
CME	Continuing Medical Education
CT	computed tomography
DEXA	dual-energy x-ray absorptiometry
DPA	dual-photon absorptiometry
ECG	electrocardiogram
FDA	US Food and Drug Administration
K-wire	Kirschner wire
MMA	methylmethacrylate
MR	magnetic resonance
NR	nerve root
PMMA	polymethylmethacrylate
PV	percutaneous vertebroplasty
QCT	quantitative computed tomography
SPA	single-photon absorptiometry
STIR	short tau inversion recovery
VCFs	vertebral compression fractures
VH	vertebral hemangioma

Appendix I

Standard for the Performance of Percutaneous Vertebroplasty*

[This standard (Res. 14, which became effective on January 1, 2001, has been included in its unaltered entirety. However, it should be noted that there are some errors in reference citations that are undergoing correction.]

The American College of Radiology, with more than 30,000 members, is the principal organization of radiologists, radiation oncologists, and clinical medical physicists in the United States. The College is a nonprofit professional society whose primary purposes are to advance the science of radiology, improve radiologic services to the patient, study the socioeconomic aspects of the practice of radiology, and encourage continuing education for radiologists, radiation oncologist, medical physicists, and persons practicing in allied professional fields.

The American College of Radiology will periodically define new standards for radiologic practice to help advance the science of radiology and to improve the quality of service to patients throughout the United States. Existing standards will be reviewed for revision or renewal, as appropriate, on their fifth anniversary or sooner, if indicated.

Each standard, representing a policy statement by the College, has undergone a thorough consensus process in which it has been subjected to extensive review, requiring the approval of the Commission on Standards and Accreditation as well as the ACR Board of Chancellors, the ACR Council Steering Committee, and the

ACR Council. The standards recognize that the safe and effective use of diagnostic and therapeutic radiology requires specific training, skills, and techniques, as described in each document.

Reproduction or modification of the published standard by those entities not providing these services is not authorized.

The standards of the American College of Radiology (ACR) are not rules, but are guidelines that attempt to define principles of practice which should generally produce high-quality radiological care. The physician and medical physicist may modify an existing standard as determined by the individual patient and available resources. Adherence to ACR standards will not assure a successful outcome in every situation. The standards should not be deemed inclusive of all proper methods of care or exclusive of other methods of care reasonably directed to obtaining the same results. The standards are not intended to establish a legal standard of care or conduct, and deviation from a standard does not, in and of itself, indicate or imply that such medical practice is below an acceptable level of care. The ultimate judgment regarding the propriety of any specific procedure or course of conduct must be made by the physician and medical physicist in light of all circumstances presented by the individual situation.

Standard for the Performance of Percutaneous Vertebroplasty

Developed by a collaborative panel of the American College of Radiology, the American Society of Neuroradiology, the American Society of Interventional and Therapeutic Neuroradiology, and the American Society of Spine Radiology.

I. Introduction

This Standard for the Performance of Percutaneous Vertebroplasty was devloped by a consensus of recognized pioneers of the technique in the United States. Physicians from the fields of interventional neuroradiology, musculoskeletal radiology, neurosurgery, and orthopedic surgery participated in the development process. A thorough review of the literature was performed. When published data were felt to be inadequate, data from the expert panel members' own quality assurance programs were used to supplement. Thresholds for quality assurance were difficult to set due to the relative paucity of data and lack of uniform reporting of clinical outcomes and complications.

Percutaneous vertebroplasy is being performed with rapidly increasing frequency in the United States. We anticipate that more data regarding outcomes and complications will be collected and published in the near future. Therefore, we recommend that this standard be reviewed and, if necessary, revised within the next 24 months in order to remain current with this rapidly progressing technique.

Developed by Deramond and colleagues in France in the late 1980s (1), percutaneous vertebroplasty entails injection of polymethylmethacrylate (PMMA) cement into the collapsed vertebra. Although this procedure does not reexpand the collapsed vertebra, reinforcing and stabilizing the fracture seems to alleviate pain.

Radiologic imaging has been a critical part of percutaneous vertebroplasty from its inception. Most procedures are performed utilizing fluoroscopic guidance for needle placement and to monitor cement injection. The use of computed tomography (CT) has also been described for these purposes.

Percutaneous vertebroplasty is an established, safe, and effective procedure for selected patients. Extensive experience documents the safety and efficacy of this procedure (1–20). As with any invasive procedure, the patient is most likely to benefit when the procedure is performed in an appropriate environment by qualified physicians.

II. Overview

Vertebral compression fractures are a common and often debilitating complication of osteoporosis (21–25). Although most fractures heal within a few weeks or months, a minority of patients continue to suffer pain that does not respond to conservative therapy (26,27). Vertebral compression fractures are a leading cause of nursing home admission. Open surgical fixation is rarely employed to treat these fractures. The poor quality of bone at the adjacent unfractured levels does not provide a good anchor for surgical hardware, and the advanced age of most affected patients increases the risk of major surgery.

Initial success with percutaneous vertebroplasty for treatment of aggressive hemangiomas (1,2) and osteolytic neoplasms (3,4) led to extension of the indications to include osteoporotic compression fractures refractory to medical therapy (5–19).

III. Indications and Contraindications

A. Indications

1. Painful osteoporotic vertebral compression fracture(s) refractory to medical therapy. Failure of medical therapy is defined as minimal or no pain relief with the administra-

tion of physician-prescribed analgesics or achievement of adequate pain relief only with narcotic dosages that induce excessive and intolerable sedation, confusion, or constipation. Associated major disability such as inability to walk, transfer, or perform activities of daily living is almost always present.

2. Painful vertebral fracture or severe osteolysis with impending fracture related to benign or malignant tumor, such as hemangioma, myeloma, or metastasis.
3. Painful vertebral fracture associated with osteonecrosis (Kummell's disease).
4. Unstable compression fracture with demonstration of movement at the wedge deformity.
5. Patients with multiple compression deformities resulting from osteoporotic collapse for whom further collapse would likely result in pulmonary compromise, gastrointestinal tract dysfunction, or altered center of gravity with associated increased risk of falling as a result of deformity of the spine.
6. Chronic traumatic fractures in normal bone with nonunion of fracture fragments or internal cystic changes.

B. Absolute Contraindications

1. Asymptomatic stable fracture.
2. Patient clearly improving on medical therapy.
3. Prophylaxis in osteopenic patients with no evidence of acute fracture.
4. Osteomyelitis of target vertebra.
5. Acute traumatic fracture of nonosteoporotic vertebra.
6. Uncorrectable coagulopathy or hemorrhagic diathesis.
7. Allergy to any component required for the procedure.

C. Relative Contraindications

1. Radicular pain or radiculopathy, significantly in excess of vertebral pain, caused by a compressive syndrome unrelated to vertebral body collapse. In such circumstances, preoperative vertebroplasty may be indicated if a spinal destabilization procedure is planned.
2. Retropulsion of fracture fragment causing significant spinal canal compromise.
3. Tumor extension into the epidural space with significant spinal canal compromise.
4. Severe vertebral body collapse.
5. Stable fracture without pain and known to be more than 2 years old.
6. Treatment of more than three levels performed at one time.

The threshold for these indications is 95%. When fewer than 95% of the procedures are for these indications, the institution should review the process of patient selection.

IV. Qualifications and Responsibilities of Personnel

A. Physician

1. In general, the requirements for the performance of percutaneous vertebroplasty (see Section IV.A.3) may be met by adhering to the recommendations listed below:

    a. Certification in Radiology or Diagnostic Radiology by the American Board of Radiology, the American Osteopathic Board of Radiology, or the Royal College of Physicians and Surgeons of Canada.

    and

    b. Completion of an Accreditation Council for Graduate Medical Education (ACGME) accredited residency or fellowship program that included 6 months training in cross-sectional imaging, including CT and MR imaging, and 4 months training in image-guided interventional radiological techniques including percutaneous vertebroplasty, biopsy and drainage procedures, and vascular embolization. This must include performance (under the supervision of a qualified physician) of at least 10 percutaneous vertebroplasties with acceptable success and complication rates documented by a log of cases performed as described in this document (see Section VII.C).

    Physicians whose residency or fellowship training did not include the above-described experience with percutaneous vertebroplasty may be considered as satisfying the qualifications for this procedure if they meet all other requirements and have performed at least 10 percutaneous vertebroplasties with acceptable success and complication rates documented by a log of cases performed as described in this document (see Section VII.C).

2. In the absence of appropriate ACGME approved residency or fellowship training (as listed in Section IV.A.1.a above) or other postgraduate training that included comparable instruction and experience, physicians may meet the requirements listed in Section IV.A.1 by adhering to the following recommendations:

    a. Documentation of "hands-on" training in the performance of percutaneous vertebroplasty.

    and

b. Performance and completion of at least two successful and uncomplicated percutaneous vertebroplasty procedures as principal operator under the supervision of an on-site, qualified physician with acceptable success and complication rates (see Section VII.C).

c. Substantiation in writing by the Director of the Department of Radiology, the Chief of the Medical Staff, or the Chair of the Credentials Committee of the institution in which the procedures were performed that the physician is familiar with all of the following:

   1. Indications and contraindications for percutaneous vertebroplasty.
   2. Preprocedural assessment and intraprocedural monitoring of the patient.
   3. Appropriate use and operation of fluoroscopic and radiographic equipment, digital subtraction systems, and other electronic imaging systems.
   4. Principles of radiation protection, hazards of radiation exposure to the patient and the radiologic personnel, and radiation monitoring requirements.
   5. Anatomy, physiology, and pathophysiology of the spine, spinal cord, and nerve roots.
   6. Pharmacology of contrast agents and of polymethyl methacrylate and recognition and treatment of adverse reactions to these substances.
   7. Technical aspects of performing this procedure.
   8. Postprocedural patient management, particularly the recognition and initial management of procedural complications.

3. Certain fundamental knowledge and skills are required for the appropriate application and safe performance of percutaneous vertebroplasty:

a. In addition to a basic understanding of spinal anatomy, physiology, and pathophysiology, the physician must have sufficient knowledge of the clinical and imaging evaluation of patients with spinal disorders to determine those for whom percutaneous vertebroplasty is indicated.

and

b. The physician must fully appreciate the benefits and risks of percutaneous vertebroplasty and the alternatives to the procedure.

and

c. The physician is required to be competent in the use of fluoroscopy, computed tomography (CT), and magnetic resonance imaging (MRI); modalities employed to evaluate potential patients and to guide the percutaneous vertebroplasty procedure.

and
d. Operator should be able to recognize, interpret, and act immediately on image findings.

and
e. The physician must have the ability, skills, and knowledge to evaluate the patient's clinical status and to identify those patients who might be at increased risk, who may require additional pre- or postprocedural care, or who have relative contraindications to the procedure.

and
f. The physician must be capable of providing the initial clinical management of complications of percutaneous vertebroplasty, including administration of basic life support, treatment of pneumothorax, and recognition of spinal cord compression.

and
g. Training in radiation physics and safety is an important component of these requirements. Such training is important to maximize both patient and physician safety. It is highly recommended that the physician have adequate training in and be familiar with the principles of radiation exposure, the hazards of radiation exposure to both patients and radiologic personnel, and the radiation monitoring requirements for the imaging methods listed above.

4. Maintenance of competence
Maintenance of competence requires regular continuing clinical activity, including:
   a. Regular performance of imaging-guided percutaneous interventions, including sufficient numbers of percutaneous vertebroplasties to maintain success and complication rates as outlined below.
   b. Participation in a quality improvement program that monitors these rates.
   c. Participation in postgraduate courses that provide continuing education on diagnostic and technical advances in percutaneous vertebroplasty.
   d. The physician's continuing education should be in accordance with the ACR Standard for Continuing Medical Education (CME).

B. Medical Physicist

A Qualified Medical Physicist is an individual who is competent to practice independently in one or more of the subfields in medical physics. The American College of Radiology considers that certification and continuing education in the appropriate subfield(s) demonstrate that an individual is competent to practice one or more of the subfields in medical physics, and to be a Qualified Medical Physicist. The ACR recommends that the individual be certified in the appropriate subfield(s) by the American Board of Radiology (ABR).

The appropriate subfields in medical physics for this standard are Radiological Physics and Diagnostic Radiological Physics.

The continuing education of a Qualified Medical Physicist should be in accordance with the ACR Standard for Continuing Medical Education (CME).

C. Radiological Technologist

The technologist, together with the physician and the nursing personnel, should have responsibility for patient comfort. The technologist should be able to prepare and position the patient for the vertebroplasty procedure, and together with the nurse, monitor the patient during the procedure. The technologist should obtain the imaging data in a manner prescribed by the supervising physician. The technologist should also perform regular quality control testing of the equipment under the supervision of the medical physicist.

The technologist should have documented training and experience in the percutaneous vertebroplasty procedure or similar interventional procedures and be certified by the American Registry of Radiologic Technologists (ARRT) or have an unrestricted state license.

D. Nursing Services

Nursing services are an integral part of the team for pre- and postprocedural patient management and education and may assist the physician in monitoring the patient during the percutaneous vertebroplasty procedure.

V. Specifications of the Procedure

A. Technical Requirements

There are several technical requirements that are necessary to ensure safe and successful percutaneous vertebroplasties. These include adequate institutional facilities, imaging and monitoring equipment, and support personnel. The following are minimum facility requirements for any institution in which percutaneous vertebroplasty is to be performed:

1. A procedure suite large enough to allow easy transfer of the patient from bed to procedural table with sufficient space for appropriate positioning of patient monitoring equipment,

anesthesia equipment, respirators, etc. There should be adequate space for the operating team to work unencumbered on either side of the patient and for the circulation of other staff within the room without contaminating the sterile conditions.

2. A high-resolution image intensifier and video system with adequate shielding capable of rapid imaging in orthogonal planes and capabilities for permanent image recording is essential. Imaging findings are acquired and stored either on conventional film or digitally on computerized storage media. Imaging and image recording must be consistent with the as low as reasonably achievable (ALARA) radiation safety guidelines. Operator should be able to recognize, interpret, and act immediately on image finding.

3. Immediate access to CT and MR imaging is necessary to allow evaluation of potential complications. This may be particularly desirable if percutaneous vertebroplasty is planned in patients with osteolytic vertebral metastasis and/or with significant preexisting spinal canal compromise. CT is desirable for evaluation of the spinal canal and intervertebral foramina if significant extravasation of cement is suspected, even if the patient remains asymptomatic.

4. The facility must provide adequate resources for observing patients during and after percutaneous vertebroplasty. Physiologic monitoring devices appropriate to the patient's needs—including blood pressure monitoring, pulse oximetry, and electrocardiography—and equipment for cardiopulmonary resuscitation must be available in the procedural suite.

B. Surgical and Emergency Support

Although serious complications of percutaneous vertebroplasty are infrequent, there should be prompt access to surgical, interventional, and medical management of complications.

C. Patient Care

1. Preprocedural care

a. The clinical history and findings, including the indications for the procedure, must be reviewed and recorded in the patient's medical record by the physician performing the procedure. Specific inquiry should be made with respect to relevant medications, prior allergic reactions, and bleeding/clotting status.

b. The vital signs and results of physical and neurological examinations must be obtained and recorded.

c. The indication(s) for the procedure, including (if applicable) documentation of failed medical therapy, must be recorded.

    d. The indication(s) for treatment of the fracture should have documentation of imaging correlation and confirmation.

2. *Procedural care*

    a. Vital signs should be obtained at regular intervals during the course of the procedure, and a record of these measurements should be maintained.

    b. Patients undergoing percutaneous vertebroplasty must have intravenous access in place for the administration of fluids and medications as needed.

    c. If the patient is to receive conscious sedation, pulse oximetry must be used. Administration of sedation for percutaneous vertebroplasty should be in accordance with the ACR Standard for Adult Sedation/Analgesia. A registered nurse or other appropriately trained personnel should be present and have primary responsibility for monitoring the patient. A record of medication doses and times of administration should be maintained.

3. *Postprocedural care*

    a. A procedural note should be written in the patient's medical record summarizing the course of the procedure and what was accomplished, any immediate complications, and the patient's status at the conclusion of the procedure (see Section VII.A.2 below). This note may be brief if the formal report will be available within a few hours. This information should be communicated to the referring physician in a timely manner. A more detailed summary of the procedure should be written in the medical record if the formal typed report will not be on the medical record within the same day.

    b. All patients should be at bed rest and observed during the initial postprocedural period. The length of this period will depend on the patient's medical condition.

    c. During the immediate postprocedural period, skilled nurses or other appropriately trained personnel should monitor the patient's vital signs, urinary output, sensorium, and motor strength. Neurological status should be assessed frequently at regular intervals. Initial ambulation of the patient must be carefully supervised.

    d. The operating physician or a qualified designee (another physician or a nurse) should evaluate the patient after the initial postprocedural period, and these findings should be summarized in a progress note on the patient's medical record. The physician or designee must be available for continuing care during hospitalization and after discharge.

VI. Equipment Quality Control

Each facility should have documented policies and procedures for monitoring and evaluating the effective management, safety, and proper performance of imaging and interventional equipment. The quality control program should be designed to maximize the quality of the diagnostic information. This may be accomplished as part of a routine preventive maintenance program.

VII. Quality Improvement and Documentation

A. Documentation

Results of percutaneous vertebroplasty procedures should be monitored on a continuous basis. Records should be kept of both immediate and long-term results and complications. The number of complications should be documented. Any biopsies performed in conjunction with percutaneous vertebroplasty should be followed up to detect and record any false negative and false positive results.

A permanent record of percutaneous vertebroplasty procedures should be maintained on a retrievable image storage format.

1. Image labeling should include permanent identification containing:
   a. Facility name and location.
   b. Examination date.
   c. Patient's first and last names.
   d. Patient's identification number and/or date of birth.
2. The physician's report of a percutaneous vertebroplasty procedure should include:
   a. Procedure undertaken and its purpose.
   b. Local anesthesia, if used, listing agent and amount.
   c. Conscious sedation, if used, listing medications and amounts.
   d. Listing of level(s) treated and amount of cement injected at each level.
   e. Immediate complications, if any, including treatment and outcome.

   Reporting should be in accordance with the ACR Standard on Communication: Diagnostic Radiology.

3. Follow-up documentation:
   a. Evaluation of long-term patient response (pain relief, mobility improvement). Standardized assessment tools such as the SF-36 and the Roland scale may be useful for both pre- and postoperative patient evaluation.

b. Delayed complications, if any, including treatment and outcome.
c. Pathology (biopsy) results, if any.
d. Record of communications with patient and referring physician.
e. Patient disposition.

B. Informed Consent and Procedural Risk

Informed consent or emergency administrative consent must be obtained and must be in compliance with state law. Risks cited should include infection; bleeding; allergic reaction; fracture; pneumothorax (for appropriate levels); and extravasation of cement into the adjacent epidural or paravertebral veins resulting in worsening pain or paralysis, spinal cord or nerve injury, or pulmonary compromise. The potential need for immediate surgical intervention should be discussed. The possibility that the patient may not experience significant pain relief should also be discussed.

C. Complication Rates and Thresholds (1–20)

While practicing physicians should strive to achieve perfect outcomes (i.e., 100% success, 0% complications), in practice all physicians will fall short of this ideal to a variable extent. Thus, indicator thresholds may be used to assess the efficacy of ongoing quality improvement programs. For the purposes of this standard, a threshold is a specific level of an indicator (e.g., complication rate) that should prompt a review. When complication rates exceed a maximum threshold, a review should be performed to determine causes and to implement changes, if necessary.

Routine periodic review of all cases having less than perfect outcomes is strongly encouraged. Serious complications of percutaneous vertebroplasty are infrequent. A review is therefore recommended for all instances of death, infection, and symptomatic pulmonary embolus.

A review may be prompted when a complication rate surpasses the threshold values outlined below (suggested thresholds are listed in parentheses):

1. Clinical complications
a. Death (0%).
b. Permanent (duration > 30 days) neurological deficit (other than radicular pain):
1. osteoporosis (0%)
2. neoplasm (5%)

c. Transient (duration ≤ 30 days) neurological deficit (other than radicular pain) or radicular pain syndrome (either permanent or transient):
  1. osteoporosis (5%)
  2. neoplasm (10%)
d. Symptomatic pulmonary cement embolus (0%).
e. Symptomatic epidural venous cement embolus (5%).
f. Infection (0%).
g. Fracture of rib or vertebra (5%)
h. Significant hemorrhage or vascular injury (0%).
i. Allergic or idiosyncratic reaction (1%).

2. *Technical/procedural complications*
  a. Failure to obtain proper informed consent (0%).
  b. Cement embolus to pulmonary vasculature without clinical sequela and estimated volume > 0.25 mL (5%).
  c. Cement embolus to epidural veins without clinical sequela and producing > 10% spinal canal compromise or estimated volume > 0.25 mL (10%).

D. *Clinical Outcomes*

1. Achievement of significant pain relief and improved mobility (osteoporosis) (80%).
2. Achievement of significant pain relief and improved mobility (neoplasm) (50%) (when treatment is performed primarily for spinal stabilization, not pain relief, this threshold would not apply).

VIII. Quality Control and Improvement, Safety, Infection Control, and Patient Education Concerns

Policies and procedures related to quality, patient education, infection control, and safety should be developed and implemented in accordance with the ACR policy on Quality Control and Improvement, Safety, Infection Control, and Patient Education Concerns appearing elsewhere in this publication.

Acknowledgments

This Standard was developed according to the process described elsewhere in this publication by the Standards and Accreditation Committee of the Commission on Neuroradiology and MR in collaboration with the American Society of Neuroradiology, the American Society of Interventional and Therapeutic Neuroradiology, and the American Society of Spine Radiology.

Principal Drafters
John D. Barr, MD, Co-Chair
John M. Mathis, MD, MSc., Co-Chair
Michelle S. Barr, MD
Andrew J. Denardo, MD
Jacques E. Dion, MD
Lee R. Guterman, MD, PhD
M. Lee Jensen, MD
Isador H. Lieberman, MD
Wayne J. Olan, MD
Wade Wong, DO

Standards and Accreditation Committee
Stephen A. Kieffer, MD, Chair
John D. Barr, MD
Richard S. Boyer, MD
John J. Connors, MD
Robert Dawson, III, MD
Robert Hurst, MD
Richard E. Latchaw, MD
Andrew W. Litt, MD
Gordon K. Sze, MD
H. Denny Taylor, MD
Patrick A. Turski, MD
Robert C. Wallace, MD
Jeffrey C. Weinreb, MD

William G. Bradley, MD, Chair, Commission
Danny R. Hatfield, MD, CSC

References

1. Galibert P, Deramond H, Rosat P, et al. Preliminary note on the treatment of vertebral angioma by percutaneous acrylic vertebroplasty. *Neurochirurgie* 1987; 33(2):166–168.
2. Deramond H, Darrason R, Galibert P. Percutaneous vertebroplasty with acrylic cement in the treatment of aggressive spinal angiomas. *Rachis* 1989; 1:143–153.
3. Weill A, Chiras J, Simon JM, et al. Spinal metastases: indications for and results of percutaneous injection of acrylic surgical cement. *Radiology* 1996; 199:241–247.
4. Cotten A, Dewatre F, Cortet B, et al. Percutaneous vertebroplasty for osteolytic metastases and myeloma: effects of the percentage of lesion filling and the leakage of methyl methacrylate at clinical follow-up. *Radiology* 1996; 200:525–530.
5. Deramond H, Galibert P, Debussche-Depriester C. Vertebroplasty. *Neuroradiology* 1991; 33(suppl):S177–S178.
6. Debussche-Depriester C, Deramond H, Fardellone P, et al. Percutaneous vertebroplasty with acrylic cement in the treatment of osteo-

porotic vertebral crush fracture syndrome. *Neuroradiology* 1991; 33(suppl):S149–S152.

7. Gangi A, Kastler BA, Dietemann JL. Percutaneous vertebroplasty guided by a combination of CT and fluoroscopy. *Am J Neuroradiol* 1994; 15:83–86.

8. Cardon T, Hachulla E, Flipo RM, et al. Percutaneous vertebroplasty with acrylic cement in the treatment of Langerhans cell vertebral histiocytosis. *Clin Rheumatol* 1994; 13(3):518–521.

9. Chiras J, Deramond H. Complications des vertebroplasties. In: Saillant G, Laville C, eds. *Echecs et Complications de la Chirurgie du Rachis: Chirurgie de Reprise.* Paris: Sauramps Medical, 1995:149–153.

10. Dousset V, Mousselard H, de Monck d'User L, et al. Asymptomatic cervical hemangioma treated by percutaneous vertebroplasty. *Neuroradiology* 1996; 38(4):392–394.

11. Jensen ME, Evans AJ, Mathis JM, et al. Percutaneous polymethylmethacrylate vertebroplasty in the treatment of osteoporotic vertebral body compression fractures: technical aspects. *Am J Neuroradiol* 1997; 18:1897–1904.

12. Deramond H, Depriester C, Toussaint P, et al. Percutaneous vertebral surgery: techniques and indications. *Sem Musculoskel Radiol* 1997; 1(2).

13. Chiras J, Depriester C, Weill A, et al. Percutaneous vertebroplasty. *J Neuroradiol* 1997; 24:45–59.

14. Lemley TJ, Barr MS, Barr JD, et al. Percutaneous vertebroplasty: a new technique for treatment of benign and malignant vertebral body compression fractures. *Surgical Physician Assistant* 1997; 3(3): 24–27.

15. Mathis JM, Petri M, Naff N. Percutaneous vertebroplasty treatment of steroid-induced osteoporotic compression fractures. *Arthritis Rheum* 1998; 41(1):171–175.

16. Cotten A, Boutry N, Cortet B, et al. Percutaneous vertebroplasty: state of the art. *Radiographics* 1998; 18:311–320.

17. Barr MS, Barr JD. Invited commentary. Vertebroplasty: state of the art. *Radiographics* 1998; 18:320–322.

18. Do HM, Jensen ME, Cloft HJ. Percutaneous vertebroplasty in the treatment of patients with vertebral osteonecrosis (Kummell's disease). *Neurosurgical Focus* 1999; 7(1):article 2.

19. Barr JD, Barr MS, Lemley TJ, et al. Percutaneous vertebroplasty for pain relief and spinal stabilization. *Spine* 2000; 25:923–928.

20. Padovani B, Kasriel O, Brunner P, et al. Pulmonary embolism caused by acrylic cement: a rare complication of percutaneous vertebroplasty. *Am J Neuroradiol* 1999; 20;375–377.

21. Cooper C. The epidemiology of fragility fractures: is there a role for bone quality? *Calcif Tissue Int* 1993; 53(suppl 1):S23–S26.

22. Cooper C, Atkinson EJ, Jacobsen SJ, et al. Population-based study of survival after osteoporotic fractures. *Am J Epidemiol* 1993; 137(9): 1001–1005.

23. Riggs BL, Melton LJ, 3d. Involutional osteoporosis. *N Engl J Med* 1986; 314:1676–1686.

24. Riggs BL, Melton LJ, III. The worldwide problem of osteoporosis: insights afforded by epidemiology. *Bone* 1995; 17(suppl):S505–S511.

25. Wasnich RD. Vertebral fracture epidemiology. *Bone* 1996; 18:S179–S183.
26. Silverman SL. The clinical consequences of vertebral compression fracture. *Bone* 1992; 13(suppl):S27–S31.
27. Heaney RP. The natural history of vertebral osteoporosis. Is low bone mass an epiphenomenon? *Bone* 1992; 13(suppl):S23–S26.

Index

A

Abbreviations, list, 195
Adamkiewicz, artery of, 14
Adenocarcinoma, metastatic, magnetic resonance imaging in, 49
Age/aging
and bone mass, 26
and osteoporosis, 41–43
Aggressive vertebral hemangiomas, computed tomography and magnetic resonance imaging evaluations of, 139–141
Alterations, in cements for percutaneous vertebroplasty, 69–74
Alternative cements, for injection, 74–75
American College of Radiology, Standard for the Performance of Percutaneous Vertebroplasty, 175, 197–210
American Society for Testing and Materials (ASTM), use of test standards to evaluate acrylic bone cements, 71–73

Analgesic effect, of calcitonin, in fracture pain, 32. *See also* Pain relief
Anatomy, of the spine, 7–23
Anesthesia
administration of, 87–88
general, for the combined computed tomography-fluoroscopy technique, 158
local, for balloon kyphoplasty, 113
provisions for equipment, 82–83
Anterior collapse, assessing, 35
Anterior spinal cord, damage to the arterial blood supply to, 14
Anterolateral approach
to the cervical spine, 93
to the upper thoracic level, 19
Antibiotics
addition to cements, 69, 71, 86–87
administration before percutaneous vertebroplasty procedures, 86–87
Apoptosis, in exposure of osteoclasts to heat, 62

Arrhenius relationship, in thermal injury, 62
Arteries
of the lumbar enlargement, 14–16
sacral, lumbar, and intercostal, 14–16
Arthroplasty, knee, blood serum levels of methylmethacrylate following, 64
Assessment, of spinal instability, 35–36. *See also* Evaluation

B

Balloon inflation procedure, 118
Balloon kyphoplasty, 109–124
Barium sulfate, opacification of cement with, 97–99
Basivertebral vein, drainage of, 15
Benign tumors, 138–149
Biochemical markers, for following intervention in osteoporosis, 32–33
Biomechanical considerations, 61–79
in addition of barium sulfate to cements, 97

Biomechanical considerations
    (*Continued*)
  in ex vivo studies of
      kyphoplasty, 121–122
  in kyphosis, 109
Biomechanical stabilization,
    65–69
Biomechanics
  basic spinal, 65–66
  of vertebral compression
      fractures, 34
Biopsy, at the time of
    percutaneous
    vertebroplasty for
    metastatic bone
    destruction, 131
Bioresorbable cements, 75
Biplane fluoroscopy
  advantages of, 84–85
  for balloon kyphoplasty,
      112–113
  for percutaneous
      vertebroplasty in
      vertebral hemangioma
      treatment, 146
  for visualizing the
      anterolateral approach
      at the upper thoracic
      level, 19
Bisphosphonates, for
    decreasing bone loss, 31
Bone augmentation, alternate
    sites for, 187–189
Bone filler devices, uses of, in
    balloon kyphoplasty,
    119–120
Bone mineral density (BMD)
  for diagnosing osteoporosis,
      26
  relationship to the
      compressive strength of
      vertebrae, 66
  and success of balloon
      kyphoplasty, 111
  values, and measurement
      method, 29
N-Butylcyanoacrylate glue,
    complementary
    injection of, in
    percutaneous
    vertebroplasty, 146

C
Calcitonin, effect of, on bone
    loss, 32

Calcium, nutritional
    requirements for, and
    osteoporosis, 26–27, 32
Calcium phosphate cements,
    74, 184
  for balloon kyphoplasty,
      comparison with
      polymethylmethacrylate,
      122
Cancellous bone, of the
    vertebral pedicle, 9–10
Cannula, removing, 101–102
Cardiovascular effect, of
    estrogen replacement
    therapy, 31
Care, patient
  postprocedural, 103–105
    in balloon kyphoplasty,
      120
    sample of orders for, 105
    standards for, 206
  preprocedural, standards for,
      205–206
  procedural, standards for,
      206
Cements
  alterations in, for
      percutaneous
      vertebroplasty, 69–71
  alternative, for injection,
      74–75
  bioresorbable, 75
  composition of, research
      opportunities, 184–186
  extravasation of
    managing with coaxial
      needle exchange, 159
    risks in neoplastic lesion
      or osteolytic lesion
      treatment, 155–156
  insertion technique
    for balloon kyphoplasty,
      119–120
    for metastases monitored
      fluoroscopically, 131
  leak of, 88–89
    into paravertebral soft
      tissues, 166–167
    into the paravertebral
      veins, 167–168
    radiculopathy as a
      complication of, 171
    treating malignant lesions,
      132
  selection of, 96–97

hydroxyapatite with
    calcium phosphate for
    kyphoplasty, 122
  volume of, issues in
      selecting, 183
  See also Calcium phosphate
      cements
Cephazolin, administration
    before interventions,
    86
Cervical pedicles, anatomy of,
    14
Cervical spine, percutaneous
    approach at, 17
Cervical vertebrae, 9
Chemical effects, of
    polymethylmethacrylate
    exposure, 64
Chemotherapy
  in multiple myeloma, 137
  sequencing of, with
      percutaneous
      vertebroplasty, 134
Classification
  of vertebral compression
      fractures, 33–34
  of vertebral hemangiomas,
      140–142
Clinical examination
  for evaluation of
      osteoporosis, 29–30
  for evaluation of spinal
      instability, 35
Clinical practice, starting,
    guides for, 175–180
Coagulation disorders, as a
    contraindication to
    percutaneous vertebra,
    129
Coaxial needle placement and
    exchange, 159
Collapse of the vertebrae, as a
    contraindication to
    percutaneous
    vertebroplasty, 129
Competence, physician's,
    maintenance of, 203
Complications
  of balloon kyphoplasty,
      121
  defined, 169
  of estrogen replacement
      therapy, 31
  due to extravasation of
      cement, 70–71

involving the pedicle,
    thoracic, 14
of percutaneous
    vertebroplasty, 165–173
    involving the pedicle, 9
    in treating metastatic
        lesions, 132–133
    in treating neoplastic
        lesions, 155–156
    in treating vertebral
        conditions associated
        with malignant lesions,
        54
    in treating vertebral
        hemangioma, 148
    potential, discussing with
        patients, 56
    rates of, for assessing
        quality improvement
        programs, 208–209
    relating to the indication for
        percutaneous
        vertebroplasty, 169–173
    of vertebral compression
        fractures, 30
Compression fractures,
    malignant, 44–50
Compression loading
    hydroxyapatite cements
        resisting, 185
    to test cements for
        percutaneous
        vertebroplasty, 72–73
Computed tomography scan
    combined with fluoroscopy
        in difficult lesions,
        156–158
    for monitoring
        percutaneous
        vertebroplasty
        procedures, 85–86
    continuous technique, for
        needle placement and
        cement injection,
        158–159
    for evaluating malignant
        lesions before
        percutaneous
        vertebroplasty, 46
    for evaluating vertebral
        hemangiomas, 138–
        139
    for guiding needle insertion,
        in the parapedicular
        approach, 20

for percutaneous
    vertebroplasty in
    vertebral hemangioma
    treatment, 146
for visualizing the
    anterolateral approach
    to the upper thoracic
    level, 19
Conscious sedation
    during balloon kyphoplasty,
        113
    during intervention, 87–88
    See also Anesthesia
Consultation, preprocedure,
    56–57
Contraindications
    absolute, to percutaneous
        vertebroplasty, from the
        standard for
        performance, 200
    to estrogen therapy, 31
    to percutaneous
        vertebroplasty, 54,
        200–201
        in malignant involvement
            of the spine, 126–129
        in a new practice, 178–179
        in sclerosis, 43
    relative, to percutaneous
        vertebroplasty, from the
        standard for
        performance, 200–201
    to surgical treatment of
        vertebral compression
        fractures, 38
Cost, of direct medical
    expenses, for
    osteoporotic fractures,
    25
Coumadin, discontinuing prior
    to surgery, 86
Courses, for instructing
    physicians in practice,
    175–176
Craig's technique
    avoiding, 14, 20, 21–22
    complications involving, in
        vertebral hemangioma
        treatment, 148
Cranioplastic, regulatory
    approval of, for use in
    the spine, 96–97
Cytotoxicity, of
    methylmethacrylate, 64,
    98

D
Decompression, surgical
    percutaneous vertebroplasty
        following computed
        tomography, 44
    in vertebral compression
        fractures, 37–38
Deep back muscles, 16
Demographics
    of benign vertebral tumors,
        138–140
    of multiple myeloma,
        134–135
Densitometry, bone, for
    evaluating osteoporotic
    metabolic bone disease,
    27–29. See also Bone
    mineral density
Devices, for delivery of bone
    cement, development
    of, 181–183
Diagnosis
    of vertebral compression
        fractures, 33–35
    of vertebral hemangiomas,
        138
Discharge instructions,
    example of, 105
Documentation, standards for,
    207–208
Drainage, of vertebral body
    veins, 14–15
Dual-energy x-ray
    absorptiometry (DEXA),
    27–28

E
Education, of physicians for
    percutaneous
    vertebroplasty, 175–176
End point, of balloon inflation,
    criteria for, 118–119
Enoxaparin, replacement of
    coumadin with, before
    surgery, 86
Epidural abscess, as a
    contraindication to
    percutaneous
    vertebroplasty, 54
Epidural involvement, in
    vertebral hemangioma,
    140
    percutaneous vertebroplasty
        with ethanol injection
        for, 143

Epidural involvement
(*Continued*)
percutaneous vertebroplasty
with glue injection for,
145–146
Epidural venous network, 14
Equipment
for percutaneous
vertebroplasty, 81–86
institutional provision of,
176–177
quality control program for
monitoring, 207
Estrogen receptor modulators,
selective, for treating
osteoporosis, 32
Estrogen replacement therapy,
for osteoporosis, 31
Ethanol, absolute
injection of, in percutaneous
vertebroplasty for
vertebral hemangioma,
143–145
for treating metastatic
lesions, 134
Etiology
of metastases to the spine,
125–126
of osteoporosis, 41–50
Evaluation
of interventions, in
osteoporosis, 32–33
of osteoporosis, 27–30
of patients for percutaneous
vertebroplasty, 41–60
criteria in metastasis with
pain, 129–131
Exclusion criteria, for balloon
kyphoplasty, 111
Exercise, and fracture rate,
prospective study, 30–31
Extrapedicular approach, for
balloon kyphoplasty,
112–113
Extreme vertebral collapse,
treatment of, 162

F
Family
including in discussion of
percutaneous
vertebroplasty with
metastatic tumors, 130

including in preprocedure
consultation, 56–57
in surgery for vertebral
hemangioma, 143
Femoral neck, osteoporotic,
prophylactic
augmentation of, 189
Fentanyl, for conscious
sedation, 88
Fever, transitory, after
percutaneous
vertebroplasty, 171
Fluoroscopy
combination with computed
tomography scan in
difficult lesion
management, 156–158
for examination before
balloon kyphoplasty,
110–111
for examination before
percutaneous
vertebroplasty, 57–58
for image guidance for
percutaneous
vertebroplasty, 84–86
for monitoring cement
addition for
percutaneous
vertebroplasty, 99, 131
for visualization of cement
in real time, 97
Follow-up, in routine patient
care, 176–177, 179. *See
also* Outcome
Fracture healing, and stiffness
imparted by cement, 67
Fracture instability, and
percutaneous
vertebroplasty, 160–162
Future directions, 181–193

G
General anesthesia, indications
for use during
percutaneous
vertebroplasty, 88
Genetic predisposition, to
osteoporosis, 26–27
Glue, complementary injection
of, in percutaneous
vertebroplasty, 145–146

Goals, therapeutic, in
percutaneous
vertebroplasty, 160–162

H
Height restoration, with
percutaneous
vertebroplasty, 68–69,
160–162
Hemangiomas, vertebral,
51–52
historic injection of
polymethylmethacrylate
for treating, 61
Hemorrhage
as a complication of
percutaneous
vertebroplasty, 172–173
risk of, after bony
punctures, 16
Hip replacement, blood serum
levels of
methylmethacrylate in,
64
Hydroxyapatite cements
advantages and
disadvantages of,
184–185
for balloon kyphoplasty,
comparison with
polymethylmethacrylate,
122

I
Image guidance, in
percutaneous
vertebroplasty
procedures, 84–86
Immunocompromised
patients, addition of
antibiotics to cement
used in, 87
Incidence, of vertebral
compression fractures in
women, by age, 41
Incidents
defined, 166
in percutaneous
vertebroplasty, 166–169
Indications
for percutaneous
vertebroplasty, 41, 53

in treating benign tumors, 125
in treating metastatic disease, 126
from the standard for performance, 199–200
for surgical treatment of osteoporotic vertebral compression fractures, 36–37
for treating osteoporosis, T-score and Z-score, 30
Inferior cervical level, percutaneous approach at, 18–19
Inflatable balloon tamp, 183
insertion of, for balloon kyphoplasty, 117
Informed consent, standards for, 208
Institutional preparation, in setting up a percutaneous vertebroplasty program, 176–177
Instruments, space for inserting, in balloon kyphoplasty, 111–112
Interosseous venous network, 14
Interventions
in osteoporosis, 30–33
in percutaneous vertebroplasty procedures, 86–105
Intraarterial embolization, for treating metastatic lesions, 134
Irradiation, and polymethylmethacrylate therapy, 53

J
Jugulocarotid vessel, avoiding, in the percutaneous approach to the middle and inferior cervical levels, 19

K
Kirschner wire (K-wire), insertion technique, in

balloon kyphoplasty, 114–115
Kümmell's disease, evaluating with magnetic resonance imaging, 43, 47
Kyphoplasty
balloon, 109–124
for height restoration, 69
Kyphosis, reversible, in vertebral compression fracture, 162

L
Laboratory studies
for percutaneous vertebroplasty, 86
preprocedure, 57
Laminectomy, in vertebral hemangioma, 149
Langerhans cell histiocytosis, secondary osteoporosis from steroid treatment for, 53
Life expectancy, and vertebral compression fractures, 109. *See also* Mortality rate
Lumbar pedicles, anatomy of, 11–12
Lumbar spine
percutaneous approach at, 20–22
thoracic thinning in, 9
Lumbar veins, drainage of, 15
Lumbar vertebrae, anatomy of, 7–9
Lung disease, restrictive, accentuation by kyphosis from compression fractures, 109

M
Magnetic resonance images
for evaluating fractures, 42–43
before balloon kyphoplasty, 111
malignant, 46–50
for evaluating vertebral hemangiomas, 51, 138–139

Malignant compression fractures, 44–50
Malignant tumors, complications of percutaneous vertebroplasty for, table, 170
Marketing, of percutaneous vertebroplasty, 177–178
Materials, for percutaneous vertebroplasty, 69–78
Mechanical stabilization, as the mechanism of pain relief in percutaneous vertebroplasty, 64–65
Mechanical tests, of percutaneous vertebroplasty cements, 71–74
Mechanism of pain relief
in malignant lesion treatment, 132
in percutaneous vertebroplasty, mechanical stabilization as, 64–65
Mediastinal sarcoma, metastatic, treating pain from, 157
Medical physicist, qualifications and responsibilities of, in percutaneous vertebroplasty, 203–204
Medical treatment, for osteoporosis, 30–33
Metastases
osteolytic, in malignant vertebral compression fractures, 44, 125
spinal, quality of life with occurrence of, 3
Midazolam, with fentanyl, for conscious sedation, 88
Middle cervical level, percutaneous approach at, 18–19
Monitoring, equipment for, during percutaneous vertebroplasty procedures, 83
Monomer-to-polymer ratio, altering, 69–70, 97–99

Mortality rate
    in hip fractures, 25
    increase in for women with
        vertebral fractures, 160
    in osteoporotic vertebral
        compression fractures,
        42
    in percutaneous
        vertebroplasty, 173
    in spinal metastasis, 126
Multiple fractures, assessing,
        in determining spinal
        instability, 35–36
Multiple myeloma
    diagnosing, 50
    in malignant vertebral
        compression fractures,
        44
    pathology of, 134–138
    percutaneous vertebroplasty
        in, after trabecular and
        cortical destruction, 156
    with vertebral compression
        fractures, 44, 125

N
National Osteoporosis
        Foundation, on bone
        mass density screening,
        29–30
Needle
    gauge of, 90–92
    insertion procedure, 88–94
        for balloon kyphoplasty,
        113–116
    size and insertion of, history,
        2
Neoplastic lesions,
        complications in
        percutaneous
        vertebroplasty
        treatment for, 155
Nerve root
    compression of, as a
        contraindication to
        percutaneous
        vertebroplasty, 129
    thoracic, proximity to the
        thoracic pedicle
        margins, 13
Neurological deficit, severe,
        association with

vertebral compression
        fractures, 43
Neurological symptoms,
        accompanying spinal
        metastases, 133–134
Nursing services, in
        percutaneous
        vertebroplasty, 204

O
Opacification, of
        polymethylmethacrylate,
        agents for, 186. See also
        Radiopacification of
        cement
Osseointegration, of cements,
        186
Osseous anatomy, 7–14
Osteoblastic lesions, as a
        contraindication to
        percutaneous
        vertebroplasty, 129
Osteoblasts, thermal necrosis
        of, exposure and
        temperature for, 62
Osteocalcin, as a marker for
        bone formation, 32–33
Osteomyelitis, as a
        contraindication to
        percutaneous
        vertebroplasty, 54
Osteoporosis
    as a cause of vertebral
        compression fractures,
        41–43
    causes of, 3
    defined, 25–26
    medical and surgical options
        for managing, 25–40
    physician's familiarity with,
        as a requirement for
        setting up a practice,
        176
    vertebral compression
        fractures in, treating
        with percutaneous
        vertebroplasty, 61–62
Osteoporotic vertebral
        fractures, complications
        of percutaneous
        vertebroplasty in, table,
        170

Outcome
    of balloon kyphoplasty, 121
    of percutaneous
        vertebroplasty
        for treating vertebral
        hemangiomas, 146–148
        in metastatic lesions,
        131–132
        in multiple myeloma, 136
    See also Follow-up, in
        routine care
Overview, of percutaneous
        vertebroplasty, from the
        standard for
        performance, 199

P
Pain
    association with vertebral
        compression fractures, 3
    and clinical fractures, 30
    diffuse, as a contraindication
        to percutaneous
        vertebroplasty, 129
    as an indication for
        percutaneous
        vertebroplasty, 41, 53,
        128–129
        in vertebral hemangioma,
        140–142
    postprocedural assessment
        of, 103–104
    transitory increase in, after
        percutaneous
        vertebroplasty, 171
Pain relief
    from balloon kyphoplasty,
        121
    and cement injection
        volume, 131
    mechanism of, 61–65
    from percutaneous
        vertebroplasty for
        vertebral hemangioma,
        143, 146–148
    from radiation therapy in
        metastasis, 133
Parapedicular approach
    as an alternative to the
        transpedicular route,
        92–93
    to the lumbar spine, 20–21

to the thoracic spine, 10
    computed tomography-
        guided, 20
Paraspinal soft tissues, 16–17
Paravertebral veins, 15
    cement leakage into, 167–168
    network of, 14
Pathology
    of benign vertebral tumors,
        138–140
    of bone metastases, 125–126
Patients
    care for, from the standard
        for performance,
        205–206
    evaluation of
        for percutaneous
            vertebroplasty, 41–60
        in vertebral hemangioma,
            142–143
    exposure to radiation during
        continuous computed
        tomography, 159
    instructions to, 57
    processing of, 81–83
    selection of
        for balloon kyphoplasty,
            110–112
        for a new practice,
            178–179
        for percutaneous
            vertebroplasty, 51–57
        for percutaneous
            vertebroplasty related to
            metastasis, 129–131
Peak bone mass, 26
Pedicles
    localization of, in balloon
        kyphoplasty, 113
    of the lumbar spine,
        anatomy of, 7–9
    size and orientation of, 9–14
    thoracic, anatomy of, 9
Pelvis, percutaneous
    augmentation of,
    187–188
Percutaneous approaches,
    17–22
Percutaneous vertebroplasty
    extreme modification for
        difficult lesions, 155–163
    history and early
        development, 1–5

Personnel, qualifications and
    responsibilities of, from
    the standard for
    performance, 201
Pharmacological agents, effect
    of, on osteoporosis, 31
Photon absorptiometry, single
    and dual, for estimating
    bone density, 28
Physician
    during continuous
        computed tomography,
        159
    during fluoroscopically-
        guided surgery, 93–94
    exposure to radiation
    qualifications and
        responsibilities of, from
        the standard for
        performance, 201–203
    training and education of,
        175–176
Plasmocytoma
    appearance of, and cement
        distribution, 136–137
    association with multiple
        myeloma, 134–135
Polymethylmethacrylate
    (PMMA)
    compounds used for
        percutaneous
        vertebroplasty based on,
        96–103
    controlled deposition of,
        challenges in, 182–183
    for percutaneous
        vertebroplasty, 1–5
    for preoperative injection of,
        to reduce hemorrhage
        in surgery for
        hemangiomas, 51
Posterolateral approach
    for balloon kyphoplasty,
        112–113
    complications of, 93
    cement leakage along a
        needle track, 2
Preoperative augmentation,
    189–190
Prevalence, of thoracic or
    lumbar vertebral
    compression fractures,
    41

Procedure
    risk in, standards for
        conveying to the
        patient, 208
    specifications of, 204–206
    techniques, 81–107
Prognosis, in hip fracture, 25
Prophylactic augmentation
    future of, 189
    and resorbable cement use,
        185–186
Prophylaxis, role of
    percutaneous
    vertebroplasty, 53
Prospective studies
    of the effect of exercise on
        osteoporotic fractures,
        30–31
    of the effect of kyphosis on
        mortality, 109–110
    of the effect of vertebral
        fractures on mortality,
        160
Pulmonary embolism,
    symptomatic, as a
    complication of
    percutaneous
    vertebroplasty, 172
Pyridinoline cross-link
    measurements,
    correlation with bone
    turnover and
    resorption, 32–33

Q
Qualifications, of personnel,
    from the standard for
    performance, 201
Quality control program
    development of procedures
        for patient education
        and safety, 209
    for equipment, 207
Quality improvement
    standards for, 207–209
    support systems for, setting
        up, 179
Quality of life
    in patients with multiple
        myeloma, 134
    in patients with vertebral
        hemangiomas, 138

Quantitative computed
  tomography (QCT), 28

R
Radiation exposure
  in continuous computed
    tomography, 159
  in dual-energy x-ray
    absorptiometry, 28
  in quantitative computed
    tomography, 28
Radiation therapy
  in multiple myeloma,
    137–138
  for pain relief with
    metastatic lesions, 133
  for treating vertebral
    hemangioma, 148
Radiculopathy
  association with benign
    osteoporotic vertebral
    compression fractures,
    43
  as a complication of
    percutaneous
    vertebroplasty, due to
    cement leakage, 171
  with malignant compression
    fractures, limitations of
    percutaneous
    vertebroplasty, 44, 132
  percutaneous vertebroplasty
    in, evaluation of relative
    contraindication to, 54
Radiographic equipment, in
  the procedure room, 83
Radiological technologist,
  qualifications and
  responsibilities of,
  standard for
  performance, 204
Radiopacification of cement
  with barium sulfate, 97–99
  for percutaneous
    vertebroplasty, 69, 70–71
Remodeling, of bone, with
  aging, 26
Remodeling space, defined, 31
Reproducibility, of dual-energy
  x-ray absorptiometry,
  28
Resorbable cements, 75. See
  also Calcium phosphate

Response letters, standard, for
  responding to requests
  for percutaneous
  vertebroplasty, 54–55
Result. See Outcome
Retropulsed bone fragments,
  identifying before
  balloon kyphoplasty,
  111
Rib fracture, as a complication
  of percutaneous
  vertebroplasty, 171
Risk
  factors in osteoporotic
    fracture, 27
  procedural, standards for
    conveying to the
    patient, 208
Robotic guidance, future of,
  for percutaneous
  vertebroplasty, 186–187

S
Sacral insufficiency fractures,
  treatment of, 188
Scintigraphy, for localizing
  symptomatic vertebral
  fractures, 42
Sclerosis, evaluation with
  computed tomography,
  43
Screening
  for osteoporosis, with bone
    mass density
    measurements, 29–30
  of physician-referred
    patients, 55
  of self-referred patients,
    55
Segmental kyphosis, for
  assessing a fracture's
  stability, 35
Selection, of patients
  for balloon kyphoplasty,
    110–112
  for percutaneous
    vertebroplasty, 51–57
  related to metastasis,
    129–131
Space, for patient and
  personnel, in
  percutaneous

vertebroplasty
  procedures, 82–83
Spinal cord compression
  as a complication of
    percutaneous
    vertebroplasty, 171–172
  as a contraindication to
    percutaneous
    vertebroplasty, 44, 129
Spinal infection, as a
  complication of
  percutaneous
  vertebroplasty, 169–170
Stability, spinal, 35–37
Standard, for performance of
  percutaneous
  vertebroplasty, 198–210
Sterile working environment,
  for percutaneous
  vertebroplasty, 82–83
Steroid use, secondary
  osteoporosis from, 42
  and percutaneous
    vertebroplasty, 53
Stiffness, restoring to
  osteoporotic vertebrae,
  volume of cement
  needed for, 67
Strength, restoring to
  osteoporotic vertebrae,
  67
Support systems
  for patient tracking, 179
  surgical and emergency, for
    percutaneous
    vertebroplasty, 205
Surgical treatment
  excision of an epidural
    component of vertebral
    hemangioma, 146, 149
  of osteoporotic vertebral
    compression fractures,
    33–38
  for vertebral compression
    fractures, advantages
    and disadvantages,
    37–38
Syringe, for inserting cement,
  88, 99
Systemic lupus erythematosus,
  secondary osteoporosis
  from steroid treatment
  for, 53

T

Technical requirements, for percutaneous vertebroplasty, 204–206

Technique
for balloon kyphoplasty, 112–121
for percutaneous vertebroplasty
in malignant lesions, 131
in multiple myeloma, 135–136
in vertebral hemangioma, 143

Thermal effects
ablation, of metastatic lesions, 134
in pain relief in percutaneous vertebroplasty, 62–63

Thoracic pedicles, anatomy of, 12–14

Thoracic spine
percutaneous approach to, 19–20
thinning in, 9

Thoracic vertebrae, anatomy of, 9

Threshold values, for triggering review from the complication rate, 208–209

Thyroid gland, avoiding, in the percutaneous approach to the middle and inferior cervical levels, 18

Tobramycin, addition of, to cements, 86–87

Toxicity, of methylmethacrylate monomer, 98

Trabecular compartment, vascular channels of, 14

Traction, height restoration with, 160–162

Transarterial embolization, for aggressive vertebral hemangiomas, 149

Transpedicular approach
advantages of, 90–91
for balloon kyphoplasty, 112–113

development of, 2
to the lumbar spine, 20–21
to the middle and lower thoracic levels, 20
for percutaneous vertebroplasty, in metastasis with pain, 131
reduced risk of cement leak in, 88, 166
to the upper thoracic level, 19

Trauma, nature of, in vertebral compression fractures, 34–35, 42

Trocar and cannula systems, for delivering cement, 89–90

T-score, for expressing bone mass density, 29

Tumors, 125–153
growth of, and exposure to heat, 62–63
relief of pain from, from percutaneous vertebroplasty, 64–65

U

Ultrasound, for measuring bone density, 28–29

Unipedicular injection, evaluation of, 67–68

University Hospital (Amiens, France), procedure development at, 1–2

University Hospital (Lyons, France), modification of technique for percutaneous vertebroplasty, 2–3

University of Virginia, introduction of percutaneous vertebroplasty at, 3

Upper cervical level, percutaneous approach, 17–18

Upper thoracic level, percutaneous approach, 19

V

Vascular anatomy, 14–16

Venography, utility of, for predicting cement leaks, 94–96

Venous system, vertebral, 14–16

Vertebrae, complete destruction of, as a contraindication to percutaneous vertebroplasty, 129

Vertebral body tests, mechanical, in percutaneous vertebroplasty, 73–74

Vertebral collapse, treating, in patients with multiple myeloma, 135–136

Vertebral compression fractures, osteoporotic, focus on, 3

Vertebral filling, amount of, for obtaining pain relief, 99–101

Vertebral hemangiomas (VH)
complications of percutaneous vertebroplasty in, table, 170
pathology and demography of, 138–140

Vertebral veins, 15

Vertebroplasty, open, 1–5

Viscosity, of cement, modifying, 88

Visualization, of cement in real time, 97

Vitamin D, requirements for, and osteoporosis, 26–27

Volume fill, in percutaneous vertebroplasty, evaluating, 66–67

W

World Health Organization (WHO), definition of osteoporosis, 26
in terms of bone mass density, 29

Z

Z-score, for expressing bone mass density, 29